POLICING PREGNANT BODIES

FROM ANCIENT GREECE
TO POST-ROE AMERICA

POLICING
PREGNANT
BODIES

KATHLEEN M. CROWTHER

JOHNS HOPKINS UNIVERSITY PRESS

BALTIMORE

© 2023 Johns Hopkins University Press
All rights reserved. Published 2023
Printed in the United States of America on acid-free paper

9 8 7 6 5 4 3 2 1

Johns Hopkins University Press
2715 North Charles Street
Baltimore, Maryland 21218
www.press.jhu.edu

Cataloging-in-Publication Data is available from the Library of Congress.

A catalog record for this book is available from the British Library.

ISBN: 978-1-4214-4763-6 (hardcover)
ISBN: 978-1-4214-4764-3 (ebook)

Special discounts are available for bulk purchases of this book. For more information, please contact Special Sales at specialsales@jh.edu.

TO KAREN, ERIKA, MAX, AND NIELS

CONTENTS

POLICING PREGNANT BODIES

INTRODUCTION

I n popular pregnancy guides, cutting-edge medical research, and pro-life propaganda, fetuses are treated as separate and distinct from the people whose bodies they inhabit. Fetal development has been mapped in exquisite detail from fertilization to birth. Pregnant people, on the other hand, are little more than incubators, and faulty ones at that, requiring constant supervision to prevent them from harming the fetuses they carry. To this day, many aspects of pregnancy are poorly understood, and many obstetricians are not trained to recognize and treat serious complications like preeclampsia and infection, especially when they occur after the birth. The combination of fervent concern for the well-being of fetuses and hostility to pregnant people has been disastrous for both.

Although our current biomedical understanding of pregnancy and fetal development is relatively new, dating back to the mid-twentieth century, many of our most cherished ideas about reproduction trace their origins back thousands of years. A great deal of what we know or think we know about procreation owes more to ancient religion and philosophy than it does to modern science. If you imagine a very old tree with very deep roots, the latest scientific understanding of procreation is like the newest green shoots on that tree. But those shoots are connected to a much vaster and older set of ideas, and these older ideas continue to influence the way we think about fetuses and the way we treat pregnant people.

For example, we still use the expression "a bun in the oven" to mean pregnancy. This metaphor appears in a text attributed to the Greek physician Hippocrates (c. 460–c. 370 BCE). It has been in continuous use for well over two thousand years. The metaphor suggests that the fetus grows in the womb the way dough rises and expands in a hot oven. It evokes a visual parallel between the swelling dome of baking bread and the growing belly of the pregnant woman. And it feels especially appropriate since baking is a stereotypically feminine and maternal activity. But the metaphor is strange as well. As anyone who has ever baked will recognize, most of the work of creating bread or buns comes before the dough is placed in the oven. Proofing yeast, mixing flour, salt, and water, kneading, letting the dough rise, punching it down, and letting it rise again—these are the steps that take effort and skill. Once you put the dough in the oven, there is nothing to do but watch and wait.

So, why did a physician two millennia ago choose a metaphor that implied that the maternal body is just a heat source and that it does no real work in making a baby? Or, the more urgent question is: why does the metaphor still make sense to us despite our vastly superior understanding of reproduction? Artists and writers compare their creations to children, and the creative process to gestation. But when we talk about actual pregnancy, most of our metaphors and similes compare the female body to a vessel, an incubator, or an oven. We describe pregnancy as passive, not active, something that happens to women, not something that women do. This mindset has consequences. An artist needs social, emotional, and financial support to create works of art. Your oven does not need social, emotional, and financial support to bake bread. "A bun in the oven" might seem like a perfectly innocent expression, just a quaint and old-fashioned euphemism for pregnancy, but it is part of a broader pattern of thinking about reproduction that we have inherited from the ancient world, and one that continues to shape the ways we treat pregnant people. Nowhere is the influence of ancient ideas about reproduction more apparent that in our contemporary debate about abortion.

On January 22, 1973, the US Supreme Court handed down its decision in *Roe v. Wade*, declaring a Texas law prohibiting abortion, and similar laws in other states, to be unconstitutional. Chief Justice Harry Blackmun (1908–1999), writing for the majority, argued that the "right to privacy" guaranteed by the Fourteenth Amendment was "broad enough to encompass a woman's decision whether or not to terminate her pregnancy." This right was not absolute. States had an "important and legitimate interest in protecting the potentiality of human life." However, the state's interest in potential life—in the fetus—could not override a woman's right to an abortion until viability, the point in pregnancy when the fetus was capable of "meaningful life outside the mother's womb." A fetus was viable at around twenty-four weeks, or the beginning of the third trimester. "If the State is interested in protecting fetal life after viability," Blackmun wrote, "it may go so far as to proscribe abortion during that period, except when it is necessary to preserve the life or health of the mother."[1] Following the *Roe* decision, abortion during the first two trimesters of pregnancy became legal in all fifty states.

Not quite fifty years later, on June 24, 2022, the Supreme Court overturned the *Roe* decision. In *Dobbs v. Jackson Women's Health Organization*, the court declared: "The Constitution does not confer a right to abortion." Justice Samuel Alito (b. 1950), writing for the majority, asserted that "the viability line [established by the *Roe* decision] makes no sense."[2] There was no reason that a state's interest in the protection of "potential life" could not begin well before viability. Each state should be able to determine for itself if and when abortion was legal. In anticipation of the court's decision, thirteen states had already passed "trigger laws" banning abortion that automatically went into effect. Most of these laws ban abortion any time after fertilization.[3] Politicians in some states have signaled their intent to introduce legislation banning or restricting abortion. Leaders in other states have affirmed their commitment to maintaining legal abortions.

In the half century between *Roe* and *Dobbs*, Americans have become increasingly familiar with images of fetuses and descriptions of fetal development. In the opening decades of the twenty-first century, we encounter fetuses in a much wider array of medical and nonmedical contexts than our counterparts in the mid-twentieth century did. We see fetuses in doctors' offices and public health messages, at political demonstrations, in movies and television shows, in advertisements, and myriad other settings. Pro-life material, which has proliferated since the *Roe* decision, is full of descriptions and images of fetuses. The purportedly human features of the unborn are used to demonstrate their personhood. And yet even when pictures of fetuses are not accompanied by an explicitly pro-life message, they almost always show the fetus detached from the maternal body, suggesting that the fetus is an autonomous individual. This is the case, for example, in the best-selling pregnancy guide *What to Expect When You're Expecting*. There is a chapter devoted to each of the nine months of pregnancy. At the beginning of each of these chapters is an image of the developing fetus in utero. The fetus is drawn in some detail, but the maternal body is just an outline. Although the text describes changes in the pregnant person's body over the course of the nine months of pregnancy, pregnancy is visually represented solely as changes in the fetus.

Seeing changes in the fetus has become a routine part of pregnancy. Sonograms (or ultrasounds) came into widespread use in obstetrical practices in the 1970s. When my brother and I were born, in 1971 and 1969, respectively, our parents had to wait until we left the womb to look at us. I saw multiple pictures of both of my sons months before they were born. Although sonograms have little medical justification, and most of the images they produce are little more than fuzzy gray shapes, expectant parents treasure these glimpses into the womb. Sonograms are so ubiquitous that they show up in depictions of pregnancy in movies and television, and they have been used in advertisements for Volvo, AT&T phone service, Valvoline motor oil, and Doritos.[4]

Medical understandings of fetal development have improved dramatically in the last fifty years. Advances in the care of premature infants make it possible for younger fetuses to survive outside the womb, pushing the point of viability earlier in pregnancy. Fetal surgery enables physicians to save the lives of fetuses with congenital abnormalities that would once have caused death in utero or shortly after birth.[5] We now know

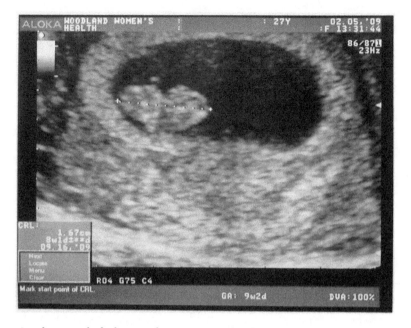

An ultrasound of a human fetus, measured to be 1.67 cm from crown to rump, and estimated therefore to have gestational age of 8 weeks and 1 day. Sage Ross, February 5, 2009. Ragesoss, via Wikimedia Commons, CC BY-SA 3.0, https://creativecommons.org/licenses/by-sa/3.0.

about the hazards that alcohol and tobacco pose to fetuses.[6] And vigorous public health campaigns have disseminated this information so widely and so successfully that any pregnant person seen drinking or smoking in public is almost guaranteed to receive disapproving comments. Many of the public health messages about the dangers of smoking and drinking alcohol during pregnancy deploy graphic images of fetuses choking on smoke or trapped in bottles of alcohol.[7] These medical developments, and the ways they have been presented to the public, blur the line between fetuses and babies, treating fetuses rather than pregnant people as patients.

As our awareness of and concern for fetuses have increased in the years between *Roe* and *Dobbs*, so too have our suspicions about and surveillance of pregnant people. In recent years, states have prosecuted women for using illegal drugs while pregnant, even if their babies were born healthy. Doctors and midwives have violated patient confidentiality to inform police of illegal drug use by pregnant patients.[8] Hospitals have tested newborns for drugs and reported findings to the police. Doctors have obtained court orders forcing women to undergo Caesarean sections and other invasive medical interventions, on grounds that such interventions were in the best interests of the fetus. In such cases, laboring women have been denied the right to make their own medical decisions.[9] Perhaps most cruelly,

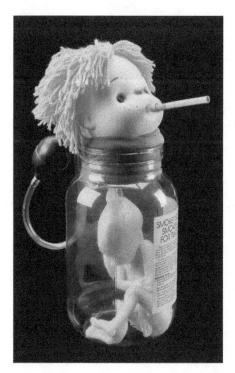

"Smokey Sue Smokes for Two" health education doll. Smokey Sue dolls were produced and marketed in England and the United States throughout the twentieth century. They were intended to illustrate the dangers of smoking to the fetus. The user would fill the jar containing the fetus with water to simulate amniotic fluid, then place a lit cigarette in Sue's mouth. As Sue "smoked," the water would become brown as it absorbed tar and nicotine. Science Museum, London. Attribution 4.0 International (CC BY 4.0).

states have prosecuted women who miscarried or gave birth to stillborn babies, even when these women had no intention of ending their pregnancies.[10] All of these trends reflect the insidious idea that the fetus requires special protection from the mother. In the interests of "protecting" the fetus, the mother's rights to privacy and bodily autonomy can be abrogated.

Since *Roe*, the maternal mortality rate in the United States has risen, and it is now among the highest in the industrialized world. The infant mortality rate has also risen disastrously. Concern for "potential life" could, in principle, lead to better conditions for pregnant or potentially pregnant people. We could, as a society, make it a priority that all pregnant people and all who could become pregnant have access to healthy food, clean water, safe housing, and medical care. We could guarantee these things to all fetuses when they are born. But we do not. Instead, we treat pregnant people themselves as the greatest threat to fetal life. To protect fetuses, we ban abortions, regulate the behavior of pregnant people, and punish them for miscarriages and stillbirths. Our beliefs, attitudes, and policies surrounding reproduction are not saving babies, and they are harming women.

The purpose of this book is to expose and untangle the roots of our ideas about procreation. This book is not a comprehensive history of pregnancy or embryology. Rather, I explore aspects of this history that can provide critical commentary on current controversies over abortion, miscarriage, and rising maternal and infant mortality rates. In chapter one, "The Tell-Tale Heart," I examine why anti-abortion advocates have chosen to privilege a beating heart as a sign of life and personhood. For over two thousand years, physicians and religious authorities have claimed that the heart is the seat of the soul and thus the most important organ in the body. Pro-life rhetoric relies on the special status of the heart in our culture. In the second chapter, "The Fetus in the Bottle," I examine the voracious curiosity to see inside the dark and mysterious space of the uterus, a curiosity that has led physicians and scientists since the ancient Greeks to observe, dissect, experiment with, and preserve dead and dying fetuses. Dead fetuses have been endlessly fascinating to scientists and physicians, living pregnant persons considerably less so. The modern separation of pregnancy from fetal development reflects this history.

In chapter three, "The Dangerous Womb," I turn to the relationship between the fetus and its mother and show that this relationship has long been conceptualized as antagonistic. Doctors imagined the womb, not as a safe and healthy place for the fetus to grow, but as a toxic environment the fetus had to survive. In chapter four, "The Secrets of Women," I show that for centuries, male writers have claimed that miscarriages are caused by women being careless or deliberately taking actions that they know will shake the fetus loose from their womb. These attitudes are still evident in our tendency to blame and punish women for poor pregnancy outcomes.

Finally, in chapter five, "Abortion and the Fetus," I look directly at the history of abortion. I examine the ways the history of abortion is used by both pro-life and pro-choice supporters to claim precedent for their positions. But I also point to the ways both pro-life and pro-choice histories of abortion have been shaped by the sources, which, until the twentieth century, are near exclusively by men. The most harmful ideas we have about pregnancy have been around for so long that they seem natural and inevitable. Examining the historical development of these ideas shows that they are not. This perspective is critical as we face the challenges of the post-*Roe* world.

The word "fetus" is taken from the Latin. It is the past participle of the verb *feto*, which means "to bring forth." *Feto* can mean "to give birth" when speaking of human or animal mothers, or "to bear fruit" when speaking of plants. "Fetus" was originally both an adjective and a noun. As an adjective it meant "fertile" or "fruitful." As a noun it meant "offspring" or "fruit." The word is simultaneously verb, adjective, and noun. It is the process of bringing a new being into the world. It is the state of being fertile, of being able to bring a new being into existence. And it is the new being itself. I would like to imagine a world in which we could recover the full complexity of the concept of the fetus, where we did not see the pregnant person and the fetus as existing separately and did not see the pregnant person and fetus as in conflict.

1

THE TELL-TALE HEART

On May 5, 2021, the Texas state legislature debated Senate Bill 8, which bans abortion "after detection of an unborn child's heartbeat."[1] The bill was introduced by one of its coauthors, Representative Shelby Slawson, a Republican from central Texas.[2] With long pauses for dramatic effect, Slawson gave a speech calibrated to appeal to her listeners' emotions as well as to claim the authority of scientific medicine. She began with a personal story:

> What seems like not that many years ago, a woman in North Texas was pregnant with her first child, an event that should have been a joyous occasion, except that it wasn't. Experiencing numerous complications, her physician told her that that little baby was not developing normally, wouldn't be fully developed, and recommended an abortion. A few days later, on a Friday, she visited another doctor, who shared that same dim prognosis of an abnormally developing baby. *But on that Friday that heart*

was still beating. And so that mom, as scared as she was, she went back to the doctor the following Monday. *And that baby's heart was still beating.* And for the next few months, the complications and those dire prognoses continued, the back-and-forth travel to the doctor continued. *And that heartbeat continued.* And then one Tuesday in May, that new mom greeted her newborn, this surprisingly normal baby, marveling at ten fingers and ten toes and wisps of red hair. And now, forty-four years and two days later, that little baby girl is standing in this chamber, *her heart beating as strongly and as rapidly as it did all those years ago,* as she lays out before you Senate Bill 8, the Texas Heartbeat Act.

At this point, Slawson was interrupted by applause. When the room had quieted, she continued: "The heartbeat is a clear and unequivocal evidence of human life, and the fetal heartbeat is a key medical predictor of whether an unborn child will reach live birth."

Slawson's speech was masterfully conceived and delivered. The word "heart" thrummed through her story at steadily increasing intervals, like a quickening pulse. Each repetition recounted a medical fact: a doctor, using a medical technology, could hear the rhythmic pulsing of a fetal heart, or the cells that would eventually become the heart. But in Slawson's story, and in the fetal heartbeat legislation she coauthored, a heartbeat is more than a medical event. A heartbeat does not just indicate that an embryo or fetus is alive, it signifies that it is *human,* an innocent and vulnerable human being, in need of all the protection the State of Texas can provide.

The juxtaposition of these two meanings of "heartbeat" has become a staple of pro-life rhetoric over the last decade, as fetal heartbeat laws have been proposed, debated, and sometimes passed in states across the country. In his wide-ranging history of the human heart, physician Sandeep Jauhar notes that in Western medicine and culture there are two different yet intertwined hearts, the biological heart and what he calls the "metaphorical heart."[3] The biological heart is a muscular organ in our chests that pumps blood around our bodies. It is a vital organ—we cannot live without it. Heart disease seriously compromises quality of life, and severe injury to the heart is almost always fatal. But the biological heart, like the kidneys or liver or gall bladder, is an organ. It is part of our bodies, but it is not our essence. The biological heart cannot think or feel or speak, any more than the lungs or stomach can.

The metaphorical heart, on the other hand, is precisely that part of us that thinks, feels, and speaks. Our language is saturated with heart metaphors. An intimate conversation is a "heart-to-heart." We feel things "from the bottom of our hearts." We know things "in our hearts." When we are sad, we are encouraged to "take heart." A cruel person is "heartless" or "coldhearted." A kind person is "bighearted" or "softhearted." Some things are "not for the faint of heart." And in the realm of romantic love, our hearts can be given, stolen, lost, broken, toyed with, treasured, aching, mended, fickle, or true. We may know that the heart is made up of muscle cells that twitch in response to electrical stimuli, but every day we speak of it as the part of us that thinks and feels. The part that makes us who we are. The part that makes us human. Anti-abortion legislation, and anti-abortion narratives like the one Slawson shared about her own origins, blur the distinction between the biological and metaphorical heart.

In this chapter, I trace both the very short history of fetal heartbeat laws (the first was drafted in 2011) as well as the very long history of ideas about the human heart and its place in fetal development that these laws tap into. The ongoing primacy of the heart and detectable heartbeat in pro-life rhetoric owes more to the cultural significance of the heart, a significance it has had since the ancient Greeks, than to any modern scientific discovery about the heart or embryology. Understanding this history is key to disentangling the scientific account of embryonic and fetal development from religious beliefs about the soul, which are tightly intertwined in pro-life arguments for heartbeat laws. Not only do pro-life advocates conflate heart and soul, as we shall see, they frequently describe the fetal heartbeat as the "voice" of the fetus in ways that effectively silence the voices and perspectives of pregnant people. After Texas S.B. 8 went into effect, Janet Porter, founder of Faith2Action, posted on the organization's website: "[T]o deny a heartbeat is to deny science. To ignore it is heartless."[4] The statement encapsulates the way pro-life advocates rely on the powerful and pervasive associations between the heart and personhood to construct arguments that claim to be both scientific and ideologically neutral. They are neither.

FETAL HEARTBEAT LAWS

The first heartbeat bill was proposed in Ohio in 2011 using model legislation prepared by Faith2Action, a Christian political group founded by prominent pro-life activist Janet Porter. On its website, Faith2Action explains: "While not the beginning of life, the heartbeat is the universally recognized indicator of life." The group notes that the heartbeat is critical in medical settings in determining whether a person is alive or dead. "In frantic efforts to save a life, we often hear: 'Can you find a pulse?' 'Is their heart still beating?' That's because science has already shown us a way to determine if someone is alive."[5] If absence of a pulse indicates that life has ended, detection of a heartbeat must indicate that life has begun. The reference to medical settings gives this "fact" the authority and objectivity associated with modern biomedicine. At the same time, because we can all feel our own pulses and heartbeats with no specialized equipment or training, the assertion that the heartbeat is an indicator of life feels like common sense.

In 2011, the heartbeat bill caused considerable controversy, not just between the pro-life and pro-choice camps, but within the ranks of the pro-choice movement.[6] Because a heartbeat, or "cardiac activity," can be detected as early as six weeks with a transvaginal ultrasound, and because few women know they are pregnant this soon, heartbeat laws effectively ban almost all abortions. Although advocates of heartbeat laws, like Porter, argued that the heartbeat signified life, six to eight weeks is far short of viability, the point at which the fetus can survive outside the womb. Twenty-four weeks is about the earliest that a fetus is considered viable, and a baby born this prematurely is highly likely to die soon after birth or to suffer permanent disability. *Roe v. Wade* established a right to abortion up until viability, and many pro-life advocates considered heartbeat laws a waste of time and effort. Such laws so clearly violated the *Roe v. Wade* decision that they would inevitably be struck down by the courts, and they could generate significant backlash against the pro-life movement. Heartbeat laws, according to some pro-life lawyers, might do more harm than good for the cause.

Despite calls for incremental restrictions on abortion, for slowly chipping away at *Roe v. Wade* rather than taking a sledge-hammer to it, heartbeat laws galvanized many anti-abortion activists and legislators. Linda J. Theis, president of Ohio ProLife Action, a group formed in October 2011 to lobby for the first heartbeat bill, said: "It's hard to be against a bill that says that once a baby's heart is beating, you shouldn't take his life."[7] Theis, like Porter, equated the heartbeat with human life. What could be heard using Doppler sonar technology was not just the rhythmic twitching of the part of the embryo that might eventually develop into the heart, but a sign of the full personhood and humanity of that "baby." Although the original heartbeat bill was defeated by the Ohio legislature in 2011, many other states drafted and debated similar bills, and several passed them. The first states to pass heartbeat bills were North Dakota and Arkansas in 2013.

The election of Donald J. Trump as US president in 2016 was followed by Trump's appointment of two Catholic pro-life judges to the US Supreme Court (Brett Kavanaugh in 2018 and Amy Coney Barrett in 2020). This emboldened pro-life advocates and tipped the balance in favor of those pushing for drastic challenges to *Roe v. Wade* rather than incremental changes. In 2018, Iowa passed a heartbeat law. In 2019, Ohio, Alabama, Mississippi, Kentucky, Missouri, Louisiana, and Georgia all passed heartbeat bills. In 2020, Tennessee and South Carolina passed heartbeat bills. None of these laws went into effect. As predicted, they were struck down or blocked by the courts. In 2021, Idaho, Oklahoma, and Texas passed heartbeat laws. On September 1, Texas S.B. 8, the Texas Heartbeat Act, went into effect, the first heartbeat bill to become law. It had, as anticipated by its opponents, an immediately chilling effect on the provision of health care to pregnant people in the state of Texas.

Before the US Supreme Court overturned the *Roe v. Wade* decision in June 2022, fetal heartbeat laws were "the anti-abortion legislative measure of choice."[8] Heartbeat laws were considerably more successful than personhood bills. Personhood bills define a fertilized egg as a person and termination at any stage after a sperm and egg have joined together as murder. While many, perhaps most, pro-life advocates believe that "life begins at conception" and would prefer that all abortions be banned, they chose, for pragmatic reasons, to concentrate on heartbeat laws. It is easier to give arguments for heartbeat bills the veneer of scientific truth. The statement that life begins at conception sounds too much like a religious point of view, and different religious traditions vary in their beliefs about when life begins—at conception, sometime during pregnancy, or even at birth. Advocates of heartbeat laws claim that their arguments about the significance of embryonic cardiac activity are rooted in scientific truth, not religious belief. This is, as we shall see, a disingenuous claim.

The use of allegedly scientific arguments in favor of abortion restrictions is part of a strategy to use secular rather than religious arguments. The Center for Human Dignity at the Family Research Council puts out a pamphlet titled *The Best Pro-Life Arguments for Secular Audiences*.[9] This pamphlet advises pro-life supporters to "ground your argumentation in science" in order to preempt "the charge that you are basing your position on faith or religious belief."[10] One of the "facts on human development" in this text is: "The cardiovascular system is the first major system to function. At about 22 days after conception the child's heart begins to circulate his own blood, unique from that of his mother's, and his heartbeat can be detected on ultrasound."[11]

It is possible to critique these arguments on scientific grounds. Many of the allegedly scientific "facts" used in pro-life arguments for heartbeat laws are either wrong or seriously distorted. For example, while it is true that the cardiovascular system begins to develop very soon after conception, it is certainly not the case that a twenty-two-day-old embryo has a fully functioning heart and a circulatory system independent of its mother's. The transfer of oxygen into the blood in the lungs is a key component of the circulation of the blood. Since a fetus is unable to breathe on its own, it relies until birth on its mother for oxygen. It cannot be said to have an independent circulatory system until after birth. Obstetricians who oppose bans on abortions after six weeks have argued that the term "fetal heartbeat" is misleading because six weeks into pregnancy (which is about four weeks from conception), the embryo does not have an actual heart.[12] Obstetricians interviewed by NPR after the Texas Heartbeat Act went into effect emphasized that what could be heard using ultrasound early in pregnancy was not, in their view, a heartbeat. Dr. Nisha Verma said,

> When I use a stethoscope to listen to an [adult] patient's heart, the sound that I'm hearing is caused by the opening and closing of the cardiac valves. . . . At six weeks of gestation, those valves don't exist. The flickering that we're seeing on the ultrasound that early in the development of the pregnancy is actually electrical activity, and the sound

that you "hear" is actually manufactured by the ultra-sound machine.

Dr. Jennifer Kerns described the "fetal heartbeat" as "a grouping of cells that are initiating some electrical activity."[13]

Supporters of heartbeat bills are not unaware of these problems. Indeed, questions about what counts as a heartbeat come up frequently during debates about fetal heartbeat laws. After Shelby Slawson told the story of her mother's pregnancy, and how her mother had refused an abortion because "that baby's heart was still beating," Representative Donna Howard, a Democrat from Austin, countered that what one could hear on an ultrasound at six weeks was "electrically induced flickering" of certain cells in the embryo, not the beat of a fully formed heart. Slawson simply said, "I don't know that I agree with that."[14] Heartbeat bills generally define "fetal heartbeat" as any "cardiac activity," a vague term that covers any discernible movement in cells or clusters of cells with the potential to develop into a heart.[15]

Beyond the question of whether what can be heard during an ultrasound examination of an embryo is the beating of a heart or the twitching of electrically stimulated cells is a more fundamental question: why attach this kind of importance to the heart? There is no inherent reason to privilege a beating heart as a sign of life and personhood. After all, the heart is only one of several vital organs, and it does not in all situations signify life. It is possible for someone to be "brain dead" but still have a heartbeat. And another sign of life—the ability to draw breath—is not present until birth. This is not a question that can be answered with recourse to science. We need to turn to history to understand the status of the heart in Western Christian culture.

HEART AND SOUL IN ANCIENT GREEK
PHILOSOPHY AND MEDICINE

"Heart and soul, I fell in love with you."

So begins the song "Heart and Soul," composed by Hoagy Carmichael and Frank Loesser in 1938. In the last eighty years it has been covered by multiple bands, used in movies and television shows, and plonked out by countless beginning piano students. The words are familiar, the sentiment timeless, and the expression "heart and soul" so common as to be a cliché. It is unlikely that Loesser, who wrote the lyrics, intended these words as a reference, even an oblique one, to Aristotle (384–322 BCE). And yet, his pairing of the heart and the soul, and his use of the phrase "heart and soul" to signify the whole person, can be traced back to the Greek philosopher.

It may come as a surprise that the concept of the soul was developed by Greek philosophers, not priests. But the soul was not at first a religious concept but rather a biological one. The soul, according to Aristotle, was the vital force that gave life to the body. Aristotle's study of the soul, and his development of the concept, was part of his study of living creatures. In his treatise *On the Soul*, Aristotle argued that all living things—plants, animals, and humans—had souls. The soul was responsible for all physiological functions. The word "organ" derives from a Greek word for "tool" because the organs of the body were the tools of the soul. For example, our soul uses our eyes to gain visual information about the world, just as a carpenter uses a saw to divide pieces of wood or a butcher uses a knife to slice meat. The faculty of sight resides in our soul, not in our eyes, just as the ability to cut belongs to the carpenter or butcher, not to the saw or the knife. If our eyes are damaged, we may not be able to see, just as the carpenter and the butcher cannot work with broken tools. Aristotle distinguished between the souls of plants, animals, and humans. In plants, which had the simplest souls, the soul enabled nutrition, growth, and reproduction. In animals, which had more complex souls, to these basic functions were added sensation and motion. Only in humans did the soul enable the highest faculty of reason.[16]

Although all organs were tools of the soul, the heart had a unique relationship with the soul. In humans, and all other animals that had hearts, the soul was lodged in the heart, like a king in his castle. In Aristotle's work *On the Parts of Animals*, he describes the heart as the "primary or dominating part" of the body, with other parts of the body "subservient" to it.[17] Aristotle believed that the heart is the source of sensation and motion, functions modern physiology ascribes to the brain and central nervous system. The ability of humans and other animals to feel pleasure and pain, and all the other sensations we perceive, Aristotle attributed to the heart and blood. Motion, too, he linked to the heart. The organ "is abundantly supplied with sinews," he noted, because "the motions of the body commence from the heart, and are brought about by traction and relaxation." The ability of humans to reason also resided in the heart. The unknown author of the first anatomical treatise on the human heart, *Peri Kardies*, composed in the fourth century BCE, expressed this Aristotelian view of the heart: "The intelligence of man is innate in the left hollow [of the heart] and rules the rest of the soul."[18]

Aristotle linked the heart not just with reason and intelligence but with character. The size and texture of the heart were linked to temperament. Aristotle describes this with reference to different types of animals, though later writers would extend it to the different character traits of human beings. "In animals of low sensibility," Aristotle stated, "the heart is hard and dense in texture, while it is softer in such as are endowed with keener feeling." Animals with very large hearts relative to the size of their bodies, like "the hare, the deer, the mouse, the hyena, the ass, the leopard, the marten," were cowardly or spiteful. The large size of their hearts allowed their blood to get colder, causing them to be fearful. Animals whose hearts were smaller were more courageous, because their more compact hearts kept their blood hotter.[19] Here we can see the origins of many of our modern idioms that link the quality of the heart to the character of the person—weakhearted, stronghearted, fainthearted, softhearted. Even the evaluation of the characters of different animals by the size and firmness of their hearts has its echoes in our culture. Who wants to be called chickenhearted? In the movie *Harry Potter and the Chamber of Secrets*, Ron Weasley looks at the swooning Gilderoy Lockhart, who has apparently fainted at the sight of the shed skin of an enormous basilisk, and comments wryly, "Heart of a lion, this one."[20] Aristotle would no doubt have shared his disdain.

Why did Aristotle link the heart and soul in this way? Isn't the brain a stronger candidate for the seat of reason? Surely Aristotle and his contemporaries would have noticed that severe head trauma can affect cognitive abilities. In fact, as we shall see, some Greek philosophers and physicians assigned the brain a more prominent role than did Aristotle. Aristotle's arguments for the primacy of the heart can be divided into three parts: (1) the heart is the first organ to form in the embryo, (2) the heart is in the center of the body, and (3) the heart is essential to sustaining life.

Let us take each of these in turn. Aristotle said that the heart was "the first of all the parts to be formed" in an embryo. In this

Galen (130–210), a towering influence in the history of medicine in Europe and in the Islamic world, adopted a somewhat different concept of the soul, drawn from the writings of Aristotle's teacher Plato (c. 425–c. 348 BCE), and a correspondingly different view of the relationship between the heart and the soul. Plato had proposed that the soul had three parts. The first controlled the most basic functions of life: nutrition, growth, and reproduction. This part was common to all living things, plants as well as animals and humans. The second part of the soul controlled motion and sensation and was possessed by animals and humans but not by plants. The third part was unique to humans. This was the rational part of the soul that enabled the higher cognitive faculties. This will seem much like Aristotle's view of the soul, and indeed Aristotle was influenced by his teacher. But the subtle difference is that Plato believed each of these three parts of the soul was housed in a specific organ. The nutritive part was in the liver, the sensitive in the heart, and the rational in the brain.[23] Aristotle had insisted that the soul (although in humans it possessed all three of these parts) was unified, not divided into three, and that the whole unified soul resided in the heart. Galen adopted Plato's tripartite soul and developed his physiology and embryology around this. The first organ to form was the liver, then the heart, and finally the brain.[24] The order of formation reflected Plato's hierarchical organization of the soul. The embryo with a liver had a nutritive soul and was equivalent to a plant. Once the heart formed and began beating, the embryo had a rudimentary form of motion and sensation, like an animal. According to Galen, this part of the soul "is located in the heart and is the source of the innate heat." It was "the living power" of the organism.[25] The brain, seat of the highest and best faculty of reason, distinctive to human beings, formed last. Galen called the rational soul "divine" and believed it did not develop until after birth.[26] The development of the other organs was complete after about thirty days.[27]

There was a lively debate about which organ formed first in embryonic development. But even Galen and others who did not accept that the heart was the first organ to form agreed that the heart appeared within a month of conception, and that the heart gave heat and life to the rest of the body. For Aristotle, the heart was the source of rational thought as well as emotions. This, too, was a subject of controversy. Galen accepted that passions and desires emanate from the heart, but he believed the cognitive faculties resided in the brain. While it might seem that such a view would make the brain and not the heart the site of the self, that was not the case. For the ancient Greeks and Romans, and for generations of Christian theologians who were influenced by them, the human ability to reason was what connected us to the divine. Our brains linked us to God; our hearts were what made us human.

That an embryo has a beating heart very early in its development is not a new revelation of modern embryology. It is a fact that has been recognized since antiquity. But modern embryology sees development from fertilized egg to blastocyst to embryo to fetus to neonate as continuous. The proponents of fetal heartbeat laws look back to a tradition started by Aristotle, which grants special significance to the moment one can detect a heartbeat, whether heartbeat is defined as that tiny pulsing point of blood you can see in a three-day-old chick embryo or the rhythmic thumping you can hear on a Doppler ultrasound in a six-week-old human embryo. This is also a tradition that makes the heart the seat of the soul and thus the essence of the person.

For centuries the notion that the heart was the seat of the soul and the source of life and vital heat held sway. The twelfth-century abbess Hildegard of Bingen (1098–1179) is best known today for her mystical visions and her musical compositions. But she was also a physician and natural philosopher, and it was in one of her scientific works that she declared that the soul resided in the heart. The soul, she wrote, "sits in the heart as in a house." Thoughts and intentions, both good and bad, emanate from the heart "as burning fire sends its smoke up the chimney."[28] In the thirteenth century, the Dominican friar Vincent of Beauvais (1184/1194–c. 1264) called the heart "the fount and origin of natural heat."[29] And Albert the Great (c. 1200–1280) confidently asserted: "Now it is agreed that the soul, with respect to the act and power of life is in the heart."[30] Mondino de Luzzi (c. 1270–1326), author of the most widely used anatomy textbook of the later Middle Ages, also declared the heart the source of the body's vital heat. He noted that the heart had the shape of a pyramid, a shape associated with the element fire.[31] Mondino refers here to Plato's *Timaeus*, in which the Greek philosopher had associated each of the four elements—earth, air, fire, and water—with a regular solid shape. Earth was associated with the cube, air with the octahedron, water with the icosahedron, and fire with the tetrahedron, or pyramid.

The Portuguese physician Valesco de Tarenta (fl. 1382–1418) compared the heart "to the sun which, standing in the middle of the planets, gives brightness to the fixed and wandering stars while, by means of light, beam, and influence, it instills in lower things the power to blossom, bear fruit, and reproduce."[32] Here Valesco drew on contemporary understandings of the influence of the sun on the rest of the cosmos. He is not declaring, two hundred years before Copernicus, that the sun is at the center of the cosmos. Rather, he takes the then-standard position that Earth is at the center and that the moon, sun, and five planets visible to the naked eye move in circles around Earth. The order of these celestial bodies, moving away from Earth, is the moon, Mercury, Venus, the sun, Mars, Jupiter, and finally Saturn. This order put the sun in the middle of the planets, with three planets closer to the earth than it and three farther away. But the sun was believed to play a special role in the cosmos, emanating heat and light. On Earth, the motions of the sun brought about the change in the seasons and made possible the growth of plants, animals, and humans.

The flourishing of anatomical dissection in the sixteenth and seventeenth centuries did little to evict the soul from its home in the heart. The great Flemish anatomist Andreas Vesalius (1514–1564) was and is widely revered for challenging the work of ancient physicians like Galen and championing the primacy of the senses and firsthand experience of dissection over the centuries-old authority of the Greeks. He was one of the first to question Galen's assertion that there are tiny pores in the intraventricular septum that allow the blood to seep from one side of the heart to the other. Yet Vesalius did not dispute that the heart was the "seat of the soul." And far from questioning this ancient belief, he approvingly cited Hippocrates, Plato, Aristotle, Galen, and the Stoics. He took the Galenic position that the brain was the seat of the rational part of the soul, and the heart the seat of the passions, the part of the soul that controls "anger or desire for vengeance and honor."[33] Vesalius, like his predecessors, located emotions like anger with the heart, as well as character traits like bravery and honor. He also believed the heart was the source of the body's vital heat. He described the heart as "the source of the vital spirit, and the seat of our natural heat and kindling."[34]

Realdo Colombo (c. 1515–1559), an Italian anatomist, challenged Vesalius's physical description of the heart. Colombo is famous for being the first European to describe the pulmonary circulation of the blood, also known as the lesser circulation. Pulmonary circulation is the movement of blood from the heart to the lungs, where it is oxygenated, and then back to the heart. Colombo's work was a critical step on the way to his student William Harvey's discovery of the circulation of blood around the entire body, also known as the greater circulation. And yet Colombo, like Vesalius, held on to the notion that the heart was the "origin of the vital heat" of the body.[35]

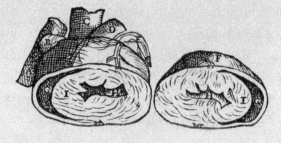

CIMA SEXTI LIBRI FIG

CIMAE FIGVRAE EIVSDÉMQVE racterum Index.

Image of the heart from Andreas Vesalius, *De humani corporis fabrica libri septem*. Wellcome Library, London.

William Harvey's discovery of the circulation of the blood, announced in his *On the Motion of the Heart and Blood* (*Excercitatio anatomica de motus cordis and sanguinis*) in 1628, and the beginnings of the modern biomedical understanding of the heart did little (at least initially) to shift the association between the heart and the emotions and character. Even Harvey described the heart as follows in his dedication of the book to King Charles: "The animal's heart is the basis of its life, its chief member, the sun of its microcosm; on the heart all its activity depends, from the heart all liveliness and strength arise."[36] As we have seen, the comparison of the heart to the sun as a source of heat and life was centuries old by the time Harvey deployed it. In his later work on embryology, he asserted, like Aristotle, that the heart was the first organ to form. Like Aristotle's, his evidence came from cracking open chicken eggs after they had been fertilized and seeing a tiny pulsing point of blood, as well as dissections of numerous animal embryos and fetuses. The heart, for Harvey, was far more than a mechanical pump.

I do not mean to downplay Harvey's achievement, which led to a radically new understanding, not only of the function of the heart, but of all human physiology. But there is ample evidence that the heart and soul remain tightly linked, even in medicine and anatomy, long after Harvey's work. This linkage persisted even among those who fully accepted Harvey's account of the movement and function of the heart and blood. What Sandeep Jauhar calls the biological heart and the metaphorical heart continued to coexist for a long time.

On December 17, 1761, a report of the autopsy of a man with an abnormally enlarged heart was read before the Royal Society of London. The report contains a discussion of the progress of the man's illness, the symptoms he experienced before his

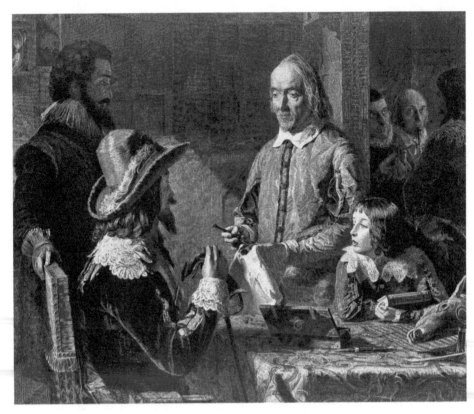

William Harvey demonstrating the palpitations of the fetal heart of a deer to Charles I. Engraving by H. Lemon, 1851, after an oil painting by R. Hannah, 1848. William Harvey, physician to King Charles I, devoted several years to the study of reproduction. The king allowed Harvey to dissect and vivisect deer from the royal hunt after the deer had mated so that Harvey could see embryos in various stages of development. In chapter 69 of Harvey's book on reproduction, *Exercitationes de generatione anima-lium* (Amsterdam, 1651), he describes how he showed the still-beating heart of a deer fetus to the king: "Having dissected the uterus, I have exposed this Punctum saliens, while it yet continued its palpitation, to the view of our late dread Soveraigne; which was then so small, that without the advantage of the sun-beams obliquely illustrating it, he could not have perceived its shivering motion." (English translation from p. 423 of the 1653 London edition: *Anatomical Exercitations, Concerning the Genera-tion of Living Creatures*.) Wellcome Collection, London.

death, and the state of his organs, especially his heart, as observed at the postmortem dissection. The man's heart "was of an enormous size, and of a very pale colour, and loose and flaccid in its texture, to a very remarkable degree."[37] The entire description of the heart focuses on observable physical properties like color, texture, and weight. This is followed by a comparison of the postmortem dissections of similarly afflicted patients. And yet, this meticulously detailed, clinical report ends with the following paragraph:

> Aristotle expressly says, that timid people, and those of cold constitutions, have large hearts; on the contrary, that the bold, and those of a warm temperament, have small ones. Nor does this opinion of that excellent philosopher seem ill founded; as women, children, and weakly men, from whom much courage is not looked for, are lax-fibred, and, consequently, more liable to an enlargement of this organ, than those of the human species, who are robust: and tense fibred, from whom a manly exertion of courage is more to be expected.[38]

More than a century after Aristotle's description of the heart's physiology had been replaced by an understanding of the heart based on Harvey's discovery of the circulation of the blood, the connections between a person's heart and the character lingered in medical writing.

Surely by the twentieth century cardiology would have gotten rid of the soul? And yet, traces of the metaphorical heart remain. The soul is not so easily dislodged from its ancient home. In 1968, surgeon Donald Effler wrote in *Scientific American*: "The heart attack is so common among professional people, executives and men in public office that it has become almost a status symbol. If all the men in these groups who have had coronary attacks were forced to retire (as airline pilots automatically are), the shortage of manpower at the top levels of government, industry, and the professions in the U.S. would cripple the nation."[39] One hears in Effler's article the echo of that eighteenth-century doctor reporting his autopsy findings to the Royal Society. Women, children, and weak men have large, flabby hearts. Such hearts beat sluggishly and are not vulnerable to the sudden crisis of the heart attack. Strong, powerful, courageous men have small, hard, tense hearts. These manly, hardworking hearts are prone to heart attacks.

Of course, Effler was not alone in his views, and twentieth-century physicians could explain the excess of heart attacks in elite men without invoking Aristotle. But the fact is, whether you cite Aristotle or invoke "Type A" personalities to explain why elite men are more likely than other groups to get heart attacks, you are wrong. Senators, surgeons, and captains of industry are not the ones most prone to heart attack. It took a massive, multiyear longitudinal study of British civil servants to demonstrate that wealthy, powerful men are *less* likely to get heart attacks than men lower down the socioeconomic ladder.[40] A janitor is more likely to have a heart attack than a CEO. And to this day, women are more likely to die of heart attacks than men, because doctors are more likely to misdiagnose women since the stereotypical heart attack patient is still male.[41] There are multiple reasons for the widespread and long-running misunderstanding of heart attacks, among both physicians and the general public. But surely one of these reasons is the long history of situating courage and intelligence, virtues particularly associated with elite men, in the heart. In this case, the metaphorical heart prevented us from seeing the biological heart clearly.

THE SACRED HEART

The heart has long had a central place in Christian culture. The word "heart" appears over eight hundred times in the Old Testament and over two hundred in the New Testament. Marjorie O'Rourke Boyle describes the heart as the "principal anthropological concept of the Hebrew Scriptures."[42] In the Old Testament, the heart is the core of a person's humanity, their spirit or what would later be called the soul. In the Old Testament, hearts can be glad or despairing; wise or foolish; righteous or wicked; yielding and submissive or hardened and stubborn; deceitful or honest. The heart *is* the person—their thoughts, emotions, desires, and actions. This is also true of the heart in the New Testament. When Matthew praises "the pure in heart" or warns that "out of the heart proceed evil thoughts, murders, adulteries, fornications, thefts, false witness, blasphemies,"[43] he, too, expresses the notion that the heart *is* the person. Goodness and evil reside in the heart. In Luke's nativity narrative, he tells us that Mary, hearing from the shepherds that angels were singing the praises of her newborn son, "kept all these things, and pondered them in her heart." Here the heart is an organ of thought as well as emotion. It also signifies interiority. In the New Testament the heart is repeatedly described as a treasure box, where one stores memories, desires, thoughts, and emotions. The New Testament heart can also be hardened or faint or troubled.

And yet, as Boyle has pointed out, there is a difference between the hearts of the Old and New Testaments. The Hebrew word (*leb*, *lebab*) in the Old Testament that is translated "heart" in English did not connote the muscular organ pulsing in our chests. According to Boyle, "There is no evidence in the Hebrew Scriptures of any anatomical or physiological knowledge of the organic heart."[44] By contrast, the Greek word (*kardia*) used in the New Testament is the same word used by philosophers like Aristotle and physicians like the followers of Hippocrates. The writers of the New Testament were men with Greek educations and cultural backgrounds, and their texts reflect both the sense of the heart as an organ that moves blood *and* the heart as the seat of that part of the soul that controls emotions and, for some thinkers, the intellect as well. When the Bible was translated into Latin, *cordis* was used for both words, and this subtle distinction was lost. Hence, since the early days of Christianity, references to the heart in both Old and New Testaments have been read as referring to the organ as understood by the Greeks. The heart, understood as the essence of a person's humanity, has been ubiquitous in Christian preaching and writing since the earliest centuries of the Church.

The *Confessions* of the Church Father Augustine of Hippo (354–430), a spiritual autobiography of his transformation from a debauched and callow youth to a Christian convert and bishop, has almost two hundred references to the heart as the essence of a person's humanity. "Thou hast made us for thyself, O Lord," he writes, "and our heart is restless until it finds its rest in thee." He describes his mother Monica as having "a heart pure in thy faith." And he prays: "Let me come to love thee wholly, and grasp thy hand with my whole heart that thou mayest deliver me from every temptation, even unto the last." In medieval and Renaissance paintings, Augustine is frequently depicted holding his heart, which is either on fire or pierced by an arrow. The fire refers to Augustine's heart being inflamed with love of God. The arrow refers to another passage in the *Confessions*, where he says God "pierced [his] heart with thy love."[45] To this day, the emblem of the Augustinian order is a heart on fire and pierced by an arrow together with an open book.

In medieval and early modern Europe, in extraordinary cases, the hearts of exceptionally pious people might bear literal traces of their devotion to God. When the abbess Chiara da Montefalco died in 1308, the nuns of her convent cut open her body in preparation for embalming. When they removed her heart, they decided to cut it open. They found an image of the crucifix imprinted on the heart and objects embedded in the organ that they identified as the instruments of the Passion, including nails, a lancet, a scourge, and a crown of thorns. When they saw Chiara's dissected heart, the nuns recalled that, several years before her death, Chiara had had a vision in which Christ appeared to her and said: "I am looking for a sturdy spot on which to set the cross, and I find here a suitable place on which to set it." It came as no great surprise to her sisters to discover that when Chiara had said she had Christ in her heart, she was not speaking metaphorically. Christ had physically placed his cross and the instruments of his Passion in her heart.[46] When Filippo Neri (1515–1595), a prominent religious leader in Rome, was autopsied, he was found to have an abnormally large heart, so large that two of his ribs had broken to make space for it. The physicians performing the autopsy decided Neri's heart had swollen to such extraordinary size because it was "inflamed by divine love."[47] When the Dominican tertiary Paola Napolitana (1572–1624) died in 1624, her body was cut open too, and her dissectors

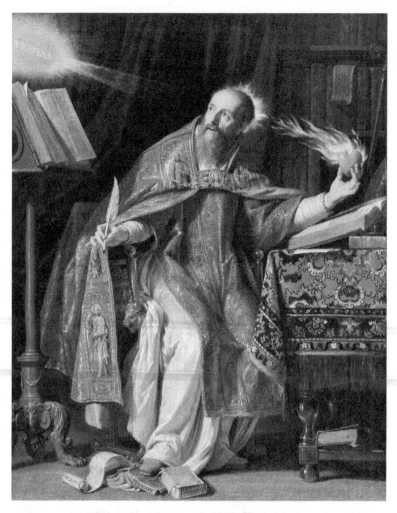

Philippe de Champaigne, *Saint Augustine,* c. 1645. A seventeenth-century painting of Saint Augustine, showing him holding his flaming heart. Los Angeles County Museum of Art, Gift of The Ahmanson Foundation (M.88.177).

found in her heart an image of the cross and a person kneeling next to it.[48]

This view of the heart was not—and is not—exclusively Catholic. Protestants like Martin Luther and John Calvin rejected the notion that sanctity might be literally inscribed on the physical hearts of holy people, and they disapproved of the veneration of the corporeal hearts of Mary and Jesus. But they accepted the idea that the heart was the seat of the soul. Reformation historian Susan Karant-Nunn has written about the importance of the heart to Martin Luther. For Luther, she writes, "The heart was the essence of each person." The heart is where we feel love and hate, joy and despair, faith and doubt. Our hearts are our characters, our selves. Luther's understanding of the heart as the "seat of personhood" is particularly evident in his preaching.[49]

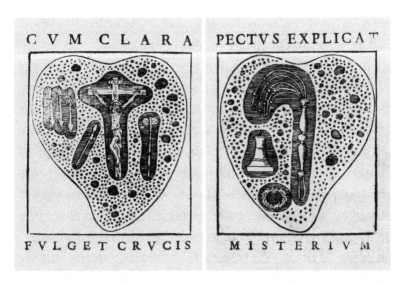

The dissected heart of Chiara da Montefalco, showing the instruments of the Passion discovered inside. Battista Piergili, *Vita della b. Chiara detta della Croce da Montefalco dell'ordine di s. Agostino descritta dal sig. Battista Piergilii da Beuagna* (Foligno: Agostino Alterij, 1640).

Luther urged his listeners to cultivate an affective, emotional relationship to God rather than an intellectual one. In other words, Christians should connect to God through their hearts, not their brains. They should embrace God in their hearts rather than engaging in rational examination of scripture and doctrine. "Where the Word [of God] remains in the heart and people diligently ponder it," Luther wrote, "there it fashions hearts which are pure, obedient, faithful, selfless, ready to help, humble and gentle."[50]

Similarly, the Swiss reformer John Calvin argued that faith and piety were not purely intellectual matters. The truth of the gospel could not be comprehended by the mind alone. In his *Institutes of the Christian Religion*, Calvin declared: "The gospel is not a doctrine of the tongue, but of life. It cannot be grasped by reason and memory only, but it is fully understood when it possesses the whole soul and penetrates to the inner recesses of the heart." Elsewhere in the *Institutes*, Calvin describes the law of God as "engraved upon our hearts."[51]

In the Anglican church, famously established when Henry VIII followed the dictates of his heart and married Anne Boleyn, the heart was also central to understandings of human nature. *The Book of Common Prayer*, first published in 1549 and containing the doctrines and liturgy of the newly constituted Anglican Church, contains multiple references to the metaphorical heart. The celebration of communion begins with the following prayer: "Almightie God, unto whom all hartes bee open, and all desyres knowen, and from whom no secretes are hid: clense the thoughtes of our hartes, by the inspiracion of thy holy spirite: that we may perfectly love thee, and worthely magnifie thy holy name: through Christ our Lorde. Amen."[52]

On into the twentieth and twenty-first centuries, Christian preachers and theologians of all denominations and political orientations have continued to speak of the heart as the seat of personhood. Five hundred years after his namesake posted ninety-fives theses on the door of the cathedral at Worms, Martin Luther King Jr. preached a sermon on the need for Christians to have "a tough mind and a tender heart."[53] In 1993 evangelical preacher Billy Graham published a best-selling book titled *Hope for the Troubled Heart: Finding God in the Midst of Pain*.[54] In 2013 the newly elected Pope Francis gave an interview in which he spoke of the need "to do the little things of every day with a big heart open to God and to others."[55] In 2018 Episcopal bishop Michael Curry began his sermon at the wedding of Prince Harry and Meghan Markle by quoting the Song of Solomon: "Set me as a seal upon your heart, as a seal upon your arm; for love is strong as death, passion fierce as the grave."[56]

THE FETUS TELLS TALES

At the close of the debate in the Texas legislature over Senate Bill 8, Shelby Slawson shared another personal story, this time about one of her own pregnancies. This pregnancy progressed far enough that she was able to see the baby (a girl) on ultrasound exams and to hear the "beautiful melody of her heartbeat." Tragically, this baby had a "severe abnormality" and died in utero. "I knew my middle daughter through the cadence of her heartbeat," Slawson said. "That sound was her song."[57] Slawson's characterization of her unborn baby's heartbeat as a song points to another troubling aspect of pro-life rhetoric: the interpretation of the heartbeat as the "voice" of the fetus. This interpretation of the fetal heartbeat is rooted in the long history of treating the heart as the core or essence of a person. Our idioms still reflect a link between the heart and speech. We can speak "from the heart" or "to the heart," and there is a "language of the heart." The technologies that allow us to hear fetal heartbeats are relatively recent, dating back to only the nineteenth century. As they have gotten increasingly sensitive and sophisticated, enabling us to hear fetal heartbeats far earlier in pregnancy than was once possible, they have also increasingly been framed as technologies that enable us to hear the "voices" of the unborn. But if technology enables the fetus to "speak," who gets to interpret what the fetus is saying? And what happens to the actual voice of the pregnant person? Amanda Nell Edgar warns that "as fetal sound gains a foothold in abortion legislation, women's voices are effectively drowned out."[58]

As I noted, the first heartbeat bill was proposed in Ohio in 2011, using model legislation prepared by Faith2Action. As part of the effort to garner support for the bill, Faith2Action recruited two pregnant women to undergo ultrasound exams combined with Doppler scanning to hear the fetal heartbeats in front of the Ohio Senate Health Committee. The women were Heather Raubenholt, twenty-four, who was fifteen weeks pregnant, and Erin Glockner, twenty-five, who was nine weeks pregnant. Raubenholt and Glockner were positioned out of view of most of the attendees while the ultrasound images of their fetuses were projected on a large video monitor in full view of all. The heartbeat of Raubenholt's fetus was clearly detectable and magnified to be audible to the entire chamber. The heartbeat of Glockner's younger fetus was too faint to hear over the sounds of Glockner's own body."[59] Significantly, the fetuses, not Raubenholt and Glockner, were described as "witnesses" and as "testifying" in front of lawmakers.[60] Glockner's fetus was hailed as the "youngest witness to ever to [sic] testify."[61] Of course, critics were quick to condemn the characterization of these public ultra-sound exams as fetal "testimony." "A fetus is scheduled to 'speak' before the [Ohio] legislature in support of the so-called 'Heartbeat Bill,'" wrote Irin Carmon for *Jezebel*, drily adding, "No word if [the pregnant woman is] allowed to talk too, or whether someone will provide ventriloquist-style commentary on the fetus's behalf."[62] After the event, and the failure to detect the heartbeat of Glockner's fetus, Carmon joked: "So much pressure! No wonder the fetus clammed up." Fortunately, "a fifteen-week-old fetus with its female incubator" was able to pick up the slack.[63] While concerns about maintaining privacy during a medical procedure in which the two women were at least partially unclothed may have dictated the decision to shield Raubenholt and Glockner, the effect of two disembodied fetuses visible on a large screen and "speaking" to the assembled crowd was also calculated to convey an argument about the independence and autonomy of the fetuses.

The ability to testify in a court of law or a state legislature implies far more than that an embryo is alive and human. It implies the ability to think and reason independently. Young children and adults with cognitive disabilities can be deemed incompetent to testify. And of course, in the United States whether a witness's testimony is considered reliable and valuable is profoundly shaped by race, gender, and class. In this historical and legal context, it is striking that the technology used to make the fetal heartbeat audible renders fetal testimony credible. Not only is this testimony produced by Doppler scanning technology, it is also mediated by people—in this case pro-life advocates—who interpret the meaning of the fetal testimony.

While the ability to hear a fetal heartbeat as early as six weeks into a pregnancy is relatively new, physicians have been listening to fetal heartbeats with stethoscopes since the mid-nineteenth century. Obstetricians used to listen to the fetal heartbeat intermittently during labor. They believed that an elevated heart rate indicated fetal distress and necessitated a more interventionist approach. In the nineteenth and early twentieth centuries, interventions usually meant forceps. By the mid-twentieth century, the intervention of choice was a Caesarean section.[64] It was, however, difficult to assess fetal well-being in this way. A normal fetal heartbeat is often twice as fast as that of an adult. Counting the beats per minute of an elevated fetal heart rate was difficult and imprecise. Further, no fetus could be continuously monitored with a stethoscope. In the late 1960s, the obstetrician Edward Hon developed an electronic fetal monitor. As historian Jacqueline Wolf points out, obstetricians presumed that the electronic fetal monitor was superior to the fetal stethoscope. It seemed so obvious that constant monitoring was better than intermittent and that the precision of machine counting was superior to the human ear that no clinical trials were ever done to compare the two methods. There is no evidence that the introduction of continuous monitoring of the fetal heartbeat led to higher rates of live, healthy newborns. The main effect of the introduction of electronic fetal monitoring was to raise the rate of Caesarean sections sevenfold.[65]

The fetoscope and the electronic fetal monitor both fostered the illusion that doctors could hear, not just the rhythmic muscular contractions of the heart muscles, but the "voice" of the fetus. It fostered the belief that the medical professionals who wielded these tools could communicate with the fetus in a way that the mother could not and that medical professionals therefore knew what was best for the fetus and even what the fetus "wanted." One obstetrician interviewed by Wolf recalled that in the 1970s he bitterly opposed natural birth and resented mothers who tried to discuss "birth plans" with him. His response is telling: "I would take the fetoscope ... put it on their abdomen and I said, 'You know I can hear your baby! Your baby is telling me don't listen to my mother! She doesn't know anything!'"[66] Having a tool that allows the physician to hear the fetal heartbeat gave the doctor access to the fetus that the pregnant person did not have. For this doctor, and undoubtedly for others, the fetoscope became a tool to reassert professional authority challenged by the women's health movement. But the way he used the fetoscope to challenge the mother's wishes indicates that he saw the needs and desires of the fetus as distinct from, and even antithetical to, those of the mother.

In addition to the dramatic rise in Caesarean sections, another unintended consequence of the introduction of the electronic fetal monitor was the rise in malpractice suits against obstetricians. Wolf explains how the introduction of the fetal monitor created the expectation that an obstetrician could accurately and reliably detect fetal distress and had a responsibility to intervene by performing an immediate Caesarean section. Unfortunately, the fetal monitor yielded no such clear indications of fetal distress.[67] In the 1980s, the lawyer, and later senator and Democratic presidential candidate, John Edwards (b. 1953) successfully sued obstetricians for malpractice after they delivered babies with birth defects, usually cerebral palsy. Electronic fetal monitoring (EFM) was key to his legal strategy. He used EFM readouts to argue that doctors had missed or ignored signs of fetal distress.[68] In the courtroom he would pretend "to be the fetus in the womb begging to be let out before it was too late."[69] Journalists described him as making "unspoken voices of injured children" heard.[70] But Wolf observes that "most, if not all, of these cases were without merit." Cerebral palsy develops in utero or affects premature infants. It is not caused by trauma during a full-term delivery.[71] As other lawyers followed Edwards's lead, malpractice insurance for obstetricians increased astronomically, and the rate of Caesarean sections rose even higher.

CONCLUSION

I titled this chapter "the tell-tale heart" after the gothic horror story by Edgar Allan Poe (1809–1849).[72] In this story the narrator plans and executes the murder of an old man with whom he lives. He carefully dismembers the corpse in a tub so there is no blood in the house and hides the body parts under the floorboards of the old man's room. The next morning the police arrive, alerted by a neighbor who heard the murder victim's final scream. Confident that he has left no traces of his crime, the narrator allows the police to search the house and then invites them into the room where the old man's body is hidden. As the narrator and the police chat pleasantly in this room, the narrator at first rejoices that he has so skillfully hidden the body of the murdered man that the police suspect nothing. However, as the conversation continues, the narrator begins to perceive "a low, dull, quick sound—much such a sound as a watch makes when enveloped in cotton." The noise, which the narrator perceives as the beating of his victim's heart, grows louder and louder. At last, the narrator, tormented by the noise, confesses his crime to the police.

Poe's story exemplifies the themes I have discussed in this chapter. The heart is the essence of the murdered man, and the heartbeat is his voice crying out from the grave for justice. Two thousand years of philosophy and religion, science and poetry, medicine and popular culture have conditioned us to think of the heart this way. Poe could have had his narrator hear scratching or raspy breathing or even a ghostly voice. But none of these would be as deliciously creepy as that eerie heartbeat, so soft at first that the narrator can barely hear it, steadily rising in volume until he cannot hear anything else. For Poe's narrator to be hearing a dead man's heartbeat, there must be something supernatural at work. But Poe's story is also ambiguous. Is the rhythmic thumping from below the floorboards real? Or is it just in the narrator's mind? Can the other characters in the story hear what he hears? This tension is never resolved.

When I read the description of the "fetal testimony" in Ohio in 2011, with the pregnant women positioned to be invisible and the heartbeat amplified to fill the legislative chamber, I thought of Poe's story. Advocates of fetal heartbeat laws insist that the rhythmic thumping we hear when a Doppler ultrasound is performed on the body of a woman who is six weeks pregnant is a person, calling out to us from the womb. But of course, not everyone hears what they hear. Despite their repeated claim that the fetal heartbeat is a "scientific fact," pro-life supporters invest the heart with spiritual significance, covertly slipping the soul back into the debate.

The spectacle created in Ohio in 2011 is an apt metaphor for heartbeat laws themselves. They render the pregnant person invisible and irrelevant. Just as Raubenholt and Glockner were removed from view (and many articles about the event did not include their names),[73] these laws erase human beings with

2

THE FETUS IN THE BOTTLE

Embryos follow a clear trajectory from fertilized egg to multi-celled blastocyst to implantation to embryo to fetus to newborn. Pregnancies, by contrast, are unpredictable and idiosyncratic. I learned the basics of embryology in my freshman biology course in college. But seeing a blastocyst under a microscope or a diagram of a six-week-old embryo gave me no clue what was happening in the body that housed them. Only when I got pregnant and read books like *What to Expect When You're Expecting* did I become aware of the physical realities of pregnancy. I'm not alone in this. There are multiple internet sites with lists of common and uncommon symptoms of pregnancy. A quick Google search of "pregnancy symptoms" turned up "Am I Pregnant? Early Symptoms of Pregnancy and When to Test;"[1] "23 Extremely Difficult Side Effects of Pregnancy That No One Warns You About;"[2] "Weird Early Pregnancy Symptoms No One Tells You About;"[3] and "10 Weird Pregnancy Symptoms That Are Totally Normal."[4] On September 3, 2022, Lucy Huber, the editor of the humor magazine *McSweeney's*, tweeted out a question: "What's your fav pregnancy symptom nobody warned you about? Mine is that my entire stomach and throat is always filled with acid."[5] She received over a thousand replies, with people reporting that their pregnancies caused carpal tunnel, sinus headaches, hemorrhoids, nasal congestion, heartburn, insomnia, sensitivity to smells, restless leg, and itchiness. Many people also commented on physical changes that lasted long after they had given birth. The repetition of phrases like "nobody warns you" and "no one tells you" suggests that the effects of pregnancy on the maternal body come as a shock to many people.

Responses to celebrity pregnancies also display a lack of understanding of pregnancy. Laura Bates, author and founder of the Everyday Sexism Project, describes how a huge number of people reacted with shock and confusion when Kate Middleton, then Duchess of Cambridge, was photographed hours after the birth of her son George still sporting a "baby bump."

> The media, both traditional and online, exploded. What was wrong with her? People *demanded* to know. Had she really had the baby? Was there another one in there? Had she got fat during her pregnancy? A quick-thinking Sky News reporter asked a midwife in an on-air interview why Kate still had a baby bump. Twitter exploded as stumped users searched for answers: "Why's Kate Middleton still fat with a bump? She's already had the baby," asked one flummoxed user. "Why does Kate's belly still look fat when they're outside holding the baby?" wondered another, concisely expressing the depth of their consternation with an added "wtf."[6]

Clearly there are large gaps in the general public's understanding of pregnancy. But why? Given that a substantial portion of human beings have either been pregnant or could get pregnant, the widespread ignorance about the physical realities of pregnancy is striking. Of course, you may not really grasp the physical realities of chemotherapy or running a marathon if you have not experienced either. But few people would be shocked if a chemotherapy patient lost his hair or a marathon runner had to ice her legs. What is so disturbing about the ignorance and misinformation surrounding pregnancy is how pervasive it is.

This is not just a matter of random men on the internet having no clue what happens to the maternal body during and after gestation. It extends to medical professionals treating pregnant women. Concern for the health of fetuses and neonates has dominated medical training and research at the expense of the well-being of their mothers. Fetal development is better understood than pregnancy, and doctors are better equipped to intervene to save the life of a fetus than they are to save the life of a pregnant person. Doctors and nurses frequently treat pregnant women as mere vessels for the fetuses they carry and dismiss their health concerns. Politicians and activists who advocate for laws restricting reproductive health care—and people who vote for such laws—downplay, ignore, and in some cases have wildly mistaken ideas about pregnancy.

Treating the fetus as a separate entity and the pregnant woman—or even just the pregnant uterus—as a passive container is not a modern development. Since antiquity, scientists and physicians have insisted on a clear separation between mother and fetus, and between pregnancy and fetal development. Further, scientists and physicians have long devoted much more attention to fetal development than to pregnancy. Until extremely recently, the main method of studying fetal development was collecting and dissecting fetal specimens, obtained through abortion or miscarriage. Dissections allowed researchers to chart, in ever finer detail, the stages of anatomical development. Pregnancy, by contrast, was studied mainly through observation of living pregnant women. Although dissections were performed on women who died while pregnant, and on pregnant animals, such dissections generally focused on the state of the uterus. When doctors and midwives treated pregnant patients, they observed a range of physical changes and problems, and they developed treatments to address these. But observation of living pregnant women lacked the precision of dissecting fetuses at different stages of development. It relied too much on the testimony of women, who were regarded as subjective, irrational, and untrustworthy. Dissection, by contrast, was objective, scientific, and certain.

ANCIENT EMBRYOLOGY

At what point in its development does a human fetus look like a human? Today, pro-life supporters routinely point out that even very young fetuses have recognizably human features. "At just six weeks," states a pamphlet prepared by the Center for Human Dignity, "the child's eyes and eyelids, nose, mouth, and tongue have formed."[7] In other words, a six-week-old fetus has a face. Fetuses also have arms and legs, fingers and toes, a penis or vagina, and internal organs. Of course, arguments for the personhood of the unborn are based on more than just the outward appearance of the human fetus. But pro-life literature and propaganda frequently use carefully composed images of fetuses, or close-ups of fetal faces or hands, to make visual, emotional claims for their humanity.[8]

The question of when a fetus has a recognizably human appearance was important to the ancient Greeks as well. Historian Konstantinos Kapparis observes that "ancient Greek doctors, philosophers and authors could not agree upon a clear and comprehensive definition of human identity."[9] Nor could they agree on when during pregnancy a fetus became a human being. The Greek philosopher Pythagoras (c. 570–c. 490 BCE) is best known today for his eponymous mathematical theorem, but he and his followers also had influential ideas about the nature of the soul. One of these was that the soul was in the seed that passed from the father to the mother in sexual intercourse. An embryo had a soul from the moment of conception, they argued, and was thus fully human starting with conception. At the other extreme, some Greeks held that a fetus was not human until it drew breath on its own. In other words, a fetus became human only when it was born. Most physicians and philosophers fell in between these two positions, holding that the embryo was human when it had developed human form, something that happened between conception and birth. There was no consensus on when a fetus or embryo acquired human form.

The philosopher Aristotle's answer was that male fetuses have human form forty days after conception and female fetuses have human form ninety days after conception. How does he know this? Because, he tells us, he has observed that a male embryo that is miscarried or aborted after forty days has human form. Female embryos, by contrast, must be at least ninety days post conception before they have definite form. Aristotle notes that miscarried or aborted embryos will dissolve rapidly, making them difficult to examine. He solves this problem by placing the embryo in cold water, which causes it to set "as if in a membrane." At forty days for males, "the embryo appears the size of one of the big ants, with all its parts evident, especially the genitalia, and the eyes very big just as in the other animals."[10] He attributes the more rapid development of male fetuses to the greater heat of the male body.

Aristotle emphasized the importance of dissection and of firsthand observation of fetuses. Dissection of pregnant animals and observation of miscarried and aborted fetuses were central to ancient investigations of embryology and remained central well into the twentieth century. Aristotle does not explain how he got access to these embryos and fetuses, or what the women who carried them thought of his investigations. We know that dissection of human cadavers was forbidden in the ancient Greek and Roman worlds, so these specimens would not have come from dissection of women who died during pregnancy.[11] Given that Aristotle claims to know the age of the fetuses he has observed, he must have obtained information about the time of conception from women. But Aristotle's observations were shaped by assumptions that we now know to be wrong. He believed males were more perfect than females, possessed of greater innate heat. This heat enabled the male fetus to take on human form more rapidly that the female fetus. For centuries, medical and scientific authorities accepted this "fact." Why didn't observation of miscarried and aborted fetuses, or dissections of pregnant animals, debunk this notion? One answer is that ancient physicians and philosophers did not really trust the testimony of women when it came to dating pregnancies. One Hippocratic writer opined that "women do not speak of the days [of pregnancy] in the same manner [as the physician], nor do they understand them."[12] If a woman's account of the date of conception matched the physician's existing theories of fetal development, he was apt to grant her credence. If it did not, he could easily dismiss her statement.

The most influential ancient writers on reproduction were the philosopher Aristotle (384–322 BCE), the Hippocratic physicians (460–370 BCE), and the physician and philosopher Galen (130–210). Aristotle was deeply interested in animals. He observed the habitats, behavior, and life cycles of insects, fish, reptiles, birds, and mammals. Whenever possible he dissected the creatures that he studied. The fruits of his extensive research were three books: *History of Animals, Parts of Animals,* and *Generation of Animals.*[13] The first two contain discussions of reproduction, and the third is devoted exclusively to the topic. Even at a remove of two thousand years, Aristotle's passionate curiosity and his appreciation for the natural world shimmer through these texts as he describes the anatomy of cephalopods, the sex lives of insects, and why mules are sterile. Accompanying his delight in the minutiae of animal life was a determination to find order and patterns in the seemingly infinite variety of living things. The central organizing principle of Aristotle's biology was the concept of the soul.

Recall that Aristotle posited that all living things—plants, animals, and humans—had souls. Possession of a soul is what distinguished the living from the non-living. A tree has a soul, but when you cut it down and make a table with the wood, the table does not have a soul. The soul is the vital force that gives life to the body. It is from the Latin word for soul, *anima,* that we get words like animate and animal. The soul is responsible for all the processes and functions of life. To continue the tree example, a living tree takes in water and sunlight, grows, and produces seeds. A table made of dead wood does none of these things. In plants, which had the simplest souls, the soul enabled nutrition, growth, and reproduction. In animals' more complex souls, sensation and motion were added to these basic functions. Only in humans did the soul enable the highest faculty of reason. To be human was to have a rational soul.[14]

The soul is immaterial, but it acts through the body. Every part of our body is a tool of our soul. We need eyes to see, but our eyes do not possess the ability to see on their own. A seamstress needs a needle to sew, but the ability to sew does not reside in the needle, but in the seamstress. The ability to see is a power of the soul. The soul uses the eyes to see just as a seamstress uses a needle to sew. If our eyes are damaged or diseased, we cannot see, just as a seamstress cannot sew with a broken or dull needle. Here then is the underlying pattern Aristotle sought. Reproduction (or any other physiological process) is a faculty of the soul. The soul can achieve reproduction in any number of different ways depending on the tools available to it. When Aristotle dissected the reproductive organs and observed the mating habits of a huge variety of animals, he was studying variations in a common phenomenon.

Aristotle posited that in animals that reproduce sexually, including human beings, the soul of the offspring comes from the father. The mother provides the material from which the body of the offspring is formed and the vessel in which it grows until ready for birth. During intercourse, males emit semen, which enters the uterus of the female. The semen contains the vital principle that causes the menstrual blood in the uterus to begin to take on the form of a new animal. This vital principle is the soul.

As the offspring takes shape in the mother's womb, it receives continual nourishment from her body, and this nourishment allows it to get larger. But the growth of the embryo is directed by the soul that came from the father's semen. This is why, when cats have sex, they generate kittens, because the male cat has implanted cat souls into the unformed blood in the female cat's uterus. When humans have sex, they generate human babies because the father has implanted a human soul into the mother's uterus. For conception to occur, the mother's uterus must contain menstrual blood for the soul to act on. Aristotle compares this process to making cheese. To get milk to "set" into cheese, you must add a small amount of rennet or a substance like fig juice to get the milk to coagulate. "Here, the milk is the body, and the fig-juice or the rennet contains the principle which causes it to set."[15] This is how the developing embryo "knows" to take on the form of a cat or a human. This is also why females, despite having the space in their bodies to generate offspring and despite providing nourishment and protection for that offspring, cannot reproduce without male input. Throughout this text Aristotle emphasizes that females are passive in reproduction, while males are active.

The soul that comes from the father is immaterial. Aristotle describes the male contribution to reproduction as "the principle of movement and of generation."[16] This may seem counterintuitive. After all, semen is a tangible, observable material substance. But for Aristotle, its materiality is only incidental. It was the immaterial soul that was conveyed with the ejaculation of semen that mattered. In fact, Aristotle asserted that the material semen did not become part of the developing embryo. The analogy he used was of a carpenter building a house. "In the same way, nothing passes from the carpenter into the pieces of timber, which are his material, and there is no part of the art of carpentry present in the object which is being fashioned: it is the shape and the form which pass from the carpenter, and they come into being by means of the movement in the material."[17]

On this analogy, the female body was a mere source of timber. In Aristotle's view, the female contribution was purely passive: she provided the materials and the workshop, but the active, creative power was male. "The male," Aristotle wrote, "is something better and more divine in that it is the principle of movement for generated things, while the female serves as their matter."[18] We can ponder the deeply ingrained misogyny that would make it possible to believe that the ejaculation of semen, which takes a matter of seconds, was a far more significant contribution to reproduction than nine months of gestation. I do not mean to suggest that semen is not essential—it is, and this was apparent to Aristotle and to people long before Aristotle—but it takes some real mental gymnastics to discount pregnancy as a purely passive and relatively insignificant part of reproduction. Modern people are still capable of these mental gymnastics. In December 2021, when the US Supreme Court started hearing arguments in the *Dobbs v. Jackson Women's Health Organization* case, Congressman Madison Cawthorn from North Carolina gave an impassioned anti-abortion speech in which he compared abortion to ripping up a Polaroid picture before it had time to develop.[19] In this analogy, the female body (the camera) has literally no role in the development of the fetus (the picture). Cawthorn used a modern technology as a metaphor for procreation, but his understanding of fetal development as something that is internal to the fetus itself and unconnected to the maternal body has an ancient pedigree.

The Hippocratic writings on reproduction are much shorter and less detailed than Aristotle's.[20] The Hippocratic physicians do not explicitly address the question of ensoulment, but like Aristotle they do lay particular significance on when the embryo has human form. They differ from Aristotle in positing that both men and women produce seed. According to the author of *Nature of the Child,* during sexual intercourse, both partners (ideally) ejaculate seed, the man externally into the woman's uterus and the woman internally into her own uterus. Sometimes the seed falls out of the uterus before further development can take place. But other times, the two seeds combine and stay in the uterus.[21] At this early stage, just after conception, the combined seeds are an undifferentiated mass of flesh. The warmth of the woman's body causes this tiny mass to thicken. The mother's breath passes into the combined seed and causes a protective membrane to form around the developing embryo. It grows in the heat of the womb like bread rises in an oven.[22] At the same time, the breath cools the flesh and causes it to articulate. By thirty days after conception, a male fetus has a recognizably human form. Because females are naturally colder, it takes the female fetus forty-two days to achieve human form.[23] As evidence, the author notes:

> Many women have aborted a male fetus a little before
> 30 days, and it showed no articulation, whereas fetuses
> aborted after, or just at, 30 days showed articulation. And
> similarly in the case of a female fetus: when the abortion
> takes place at 42 days the limbs show articulation.
> Whether the fetus is aborted earlier or later, this is when
> articulation becomes apparent both in theory and in fact:
> in a female fetus at 42 days and in a male fetus at 30.[24]

In another Hippocratic text, *Fleshes,* the author claimed to have observed more than one seven-day-old embryo. These, he asserted, had human form already. They had faces, arms, legs, fingers, toes, and genitals. This author believed that the development of the fetus from conception to birth could be divided into seven-day periods. As historian Ann Hanson comments, it is apparent that "he allowed theory to determine the age of the embryos he saw," insisting on a later date of conception for a much older fetus.[25]

The Roman physician Galen also wrote extensively about reproduction.[26] Galen begins his treatise on the formation of the embryo by complaining that "both physicians as well as philosophers have undertaken to write about the development of the embryo, without offering any evidence from anatomy for their statements."[27] Galen asserts that the best way to answer questions about the male and female contribution to reproduction, the order of formation of the organs in the fetus, and the timing of ensoulment is a sustained program of dissection. But Galen was also a philosopher, and like Aristotle, he was interested in questions about the soul. Galen's mature understanding of human reproduction drew on the work of physicians, especially the Hippocratic doctors, as well as on the work of philosophers. In terms of Galen's understanding of the soul, the most important influence was Aristotle's teacher Plato, who posited that the soul had three parts: nutritive, sensitive, and rational. In Galen's physiology each part of the soul was housed in a specific organ. The nutritive part was in the liver, the sensitive in the heart, and the rational in the brain.[28]

Galen's understanding of fetal development combined elements of the Hippocratic physicians and of Plato. Like the Hippocratic physicians, Galen posited that both men and women produce seeds and that the two seeds combine in the uterus following "successful" sexual intercourse. The first organ to form was the liver, then the heart, and finally the brain. The order of formation reflected Plato's hierarchical organization of the soul. The embryo with a liver had a nutritive soul and was equivalent to a plant. Once the heart formed and began beating, the embryo had a rudimentary form of motion and sensation, like an animal. According to Galen, this part of the soul "is located in the heart and is the source of the innate heat; . . . it is called the living power (. . .), the spirited power (. . .), the living soul, and the spirited soul."[29] The brain, seat of the highest and best faculty of reason, distinctive to human beings, formed last.[30] The development of these organs was complete after about thirty days.[31]

Our understanding of reproduction has advanced far beyond that of Aristotle, Hippocrates, and Galen. But we still debate when a fetus has a human form. And we still connect human appearance with personhood when we talk about embryos and fetuses. Pro-life advocates insist that the (allegedly) humanlike features of even very young embryos are proof that they are "babies." The importance of the humanlike appearance of embryos to pro-life arguments is illustrated by the controversy that erupted in October 2022, when *Guardian* editor Poppy Noor published an article titled "What a Pregnancy Actually Looks Like before 10 Weeks—In Pictures."[32] The article included photographs provided by clinicians from the My Abortion Network (MYA Network) showing tissue from abortions performed between five and nine weeks of pregnancy.[33] These images show blobs of white tissue, in clear petri dishes, photographed against a blue background. They resemble cloud formations, not infants. Several include a ruler to indicate the actual size of the tissue fragments. One of the MYA Network physicians, Dr. Joan Fleischman, commented that the appearance of this tissue frequently surprises physicians and medical students as well as patients. "They're expecting to see a little fetus with hands—a developed, miniature baby," she says, and that is not what an embryo that is less than seven weeks old looks like.

The response to the article from pro-life groups was swift and fierce. Monica Snyder posted a blog on the Secular Pro-Life website denouncing the photos in the *Guardian* as "biological obfuscation and misinformation." She argued that that the MYA photographs did not look human because "abortion procedures can destroy embryos beyond recognition." And she criticized the collection and visualization methods of the MYA physicians, insisting that the specimens had been rendered "artificially monochromatic," which "erased" the human features of the embryos.[34]

Writing for the Catholic News Agency, Edie Heipel claimed that the photographs were not embryos but "white pieces of the gestational sac and surrounding decidual tissue."[35] She quoted Dr. Christina Francis of the American Association of Pro-Life Obstetricians and Gynecologists, who accused the *Guardian* and MYA Network of "dehumaniz[ing] preborn human beings" by showing them as formless blobs of tissue. Heipel countered with an image of an embryo from the ninth week of pregnancy (that is, older than any of the embryos in the MYA images). Her image shows a delicate pink embryo, encased in a translucent gestational sac, magnified so that its features—eyes, nose, ears, hands, feet, fingers, and toes—are clearly visible. This embryo is not a tissue specimen in a petri dish. Rather, it floats gracefully against a black background like a miniature astronaut in a space suit. Of course, the method of preparing this embryo to be photographed was no less "artificial" than the methods employed to prepare the MYA embryos.

Some of the discrepancy between the MYA photographs of tissue in petri dishes and the images of embryos and fetuses used in pro-life material is simply magnification. There is a difference between what is visible to the naked eye and what can be seen when the embryo is viewed under a microscope. But some of the critics, like Heipel, contrasted the MYA photographs with descriptions and images of embryos that were several weeks older, suggesting (incorrectly) that embryos of four or five weeks have human form and are visible to the naked eye. The controversy sparked by the *Guardian* article recalls the debates in the ancient world about whether an embryo had human form at seven days, or thirty, or forty-two. And just like the ancient argument, the modern fixation on when an embryo has human form treats changes in the maternal body as irrelevant.

THE ANATOMY OF GENERATION

Fascination with reproduction continued into the Middle Ages and Renaissance. And as anatomical dissection flourished in medical schools, the number of dissections of pregnant women and fetuses rose dramatically. Muslim, Jewish, and Christian writers took up the subject of reproduction and expanded on the work of the ancients.[36] These writers, who included theologians, philosophers, and physicians, combined and synthesized the work of the ancients, smoothed out some of the obvious discrepancies, and adapted ancient theories of generation to their own religious views. Men of all three Abrahamic faiths believed that each human soul was specially created by God and was immortal. Most medical writers adopted the Hippocratic and Galenic position that the embryo did not have a human soul until sometime after conception. They agreed that this happened by divine fiat once the fetus had developed far enough that it had a recognizably human form. They disagreed on how long this took, although all believed males developed faster than females. When the fetus had a human form, God gave it a rational soul, and from that point on it was human. Some philosophers and theologians sided with Aristotle and argued that ensoulment occurred at conception. There were many attempts to reconcile these views, and much medieval and early modern writing on human reproduction contains elements of both positions. Medieval and early modern investigators continued to separate fetal development and pregnancy and to privilege the former in their investigations.

Although the ancient writers were widely respected, many physicians were highly motivated to test and challenge these traditional authorities. They sought to see the earliest phases of human life with their own eyes, to verify or to correct what they learned from the ancient Greeks. Historian of medicine Katharine Park argues that interest in reproduction was central to the emergence of human dissection in late medieval Europe. Anatomists, contends Park, were fascinated by the female body, especially the uterus, because this was where human life began. "The female body," Park writes, "emerged . . . as the ideal type of body, with a hidden and secret interior, the paradigmatic object of dissection."[37] Anatomists in the fifteenth, sixteenth, and seventeenth centuries displayed keen interest in the processes of conception and fetal development, and many of them dissected cadavers of pregnant women, miscarried fetuses, and stillborn infants, as well as pregnant dogs and pigs, to understand these processes better. But their interest was in fetal development, not in pregnancy. Changes to the maternal body during gestation were incidental.

Examples of investigations of human reproduction are myriad and demonstrate widespread interest in generation. In some cases, we have only brief accounts of dissections of fetuses and infants. For example, we know from contemporary reports that the Montpellier medical professor Guillaume Rondelet (1507–1566) caused a stir when he publicly dissected his own stillborn son.[38] In 1533, in Santo Domingo in Hispaniola (now the Dominican Republic), the surgeon Joan Camacho and the physicians Hernando de Sepulveda and Rodrigo Navarro dissected the conjoined twins Melchiora and Joana Balestero, who died eight days after birth, in order to ascertain whether they were one soul or two.[39] The Swiss physician Felix Platter (1536–1614) included images of the skeletons of a fetus of two months and a newborn in his *On the Structure and Use of the Human Body* of 1583.[40] Another Swiss physician, Caspar Bauhin (1560–1624), included images of fetuses of fourteen and twenty-five days in his *Theater of Anatomy*.[41] Neither Platter nor Bauhin describe how they obtained these specimens, and neither indicates that they made a regular practice of dissecting fetuses or neonates. Other anatomists, including Gabriele Zerbi, Realdo Colombo, and Volcher Coiter, described dissections and observations of multiple fetuses, stillborn infants, and babies who died soon after birth.

The Veronese anatomist Gabriele Zerbi (1445–1505), who taught medicine at the universities of Bologna and Padua, published a comprehensive work on human anatomy in 1502.[42] This book included a long section at the end on the "generation of the embryo."[43] Zerbi cites a wide range of authorities, not just Aristotle, Hippocrates, and Galen, but many medieval authors

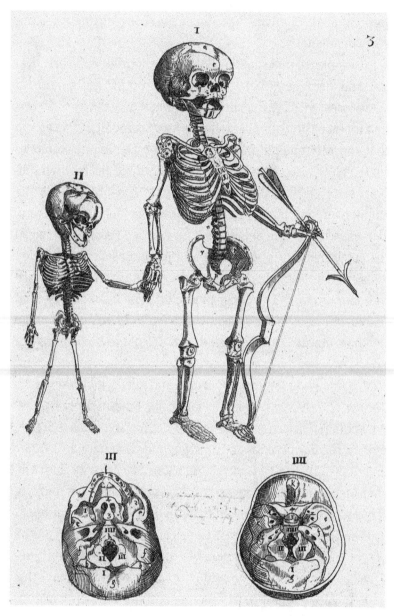

Skeletons of a newborn and a two-month-old fetus, from Felix Platter, *De corporis humani structura et usu*. Attribution 4.0 International (CC by 4.0). Wellcome Collection, London.

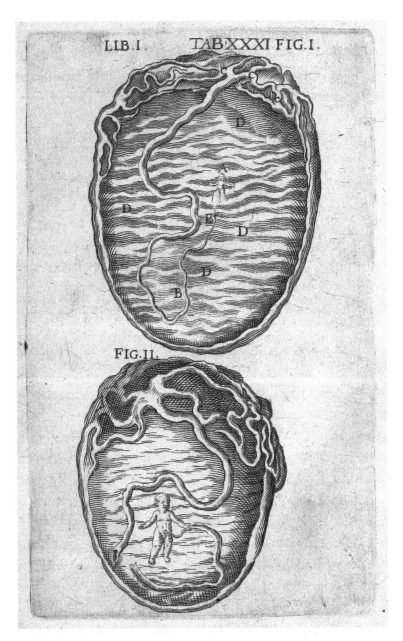

Fourteen- and twenty-five-day-old fetuses, from Caspar Bauhin, *Theatrum anatomicum / novis figuris aeneis illustratum, et in lucem emissum opera et sumptibus Theodori de Bry*, 1605. Wellcome Collection, London.

as well, including Avicenna, Averroes, Haly Abbas, Thomas Aquinas, and Albertus Magnus. His account of fetal development incorporates both Aristotelian and Hippocratic-Galenic elements. He holds, like Aristotle, that the heart is the first organ to form. He repeats Aristotle's observations of miscarried fetuses, asserting that male fetuses have recognizably human form after about forty days, females only after ninety, and that a male fetus of forty days is the size of an ant.[44] But he takes Aristotle's observations a step further. He asserts that a male fetus of forty days can sense external stimuli, something he has determined experimentally. If you prick the newly miscarried fetus with something sharp, it flinches, which demonstrates that it can sense.[45] It is not clear whether Zerbi conducted these experiments himself or whether he is reporting the findings of another author. In either case, the description of these observations and tests on miscarried fetuses is indicative of the value placed on empirical methods. They also demonstrate the ongoing interest in the question of ensoulment. The fact that a male fetus of forty days has a recognizably human form would seem to imply readiness for ensoulment. The observation that it can move and sense implies the existence of an animal soul, though not necessarily a rational soul.

Realdo Colombo (c. 1515–1559), an anatomist who taught at the universities of Padua, Pisa, and Rome, included a chapter "on the formation of the fetus" (*de formatione foetus*) in his *De re anatomica* of 1559.[46] Colombo asserted that much of what was written about fetal development was wrong because anatomists "have transferred the things they have observed in imperfect brutes to humans with great error."[47] This critique included the ancients, including "the great Hippocrates, who could not know everything by himself."[48] But it also included his contemporaries. Colombo is particularly scathing about his former friend turned bitter rival Andreas Vesalius (1514–1564). Vesalius's description of the placenta, Colombo writes, is inaccurate because it was based on dissections of dogs.[49] Throughout this chapter, Colombo touts his own experiential knowledge of human conception and generation. For example, he is able to confirm Galen's argument that the liver is the first organ to form because he has "not once but often been able to examine closely and to consider" the subject.[50] He recounts that "the great philosopher Hieronymus Pontanus" demonstrated that the liver is present in the fetus before the heart by dissecting a one-month-old fetus in front of Colombo and "an assembly of illustrious men and nobles" at the Roman Academy.[51]

The Dutch anatomist Volcher Coiter wrote *An Anatomical Treatise on the Bones of an Aborted Fetus and of a Six-Months-Old Infant*, which was first published in 1573.[52] In the introduction Coiter states that he has made sustained anatomical investigations of fetuses and children of various ages over the course of many years. As a medical student in Bologna, he obtained skeletons of children to compare with those of adults.[53] Along with some of his professors and fellow students, he examined several miscarried fetuses, including one of forty days, which he described as follows:

> The head was the size of a hazelnut and larger than the proportion of the rest of the body. The eyes bulged like a crab's; [he had] nose, ears, arms, hands, legs, feet, and separate toes; [he had] a visible penis, underneath which the scrotum [was] the size of a millet seed. The upper parts [of the body were] larger than the lower, none of the bones [were] hard, but flexible whichever way they were directed.[54]

He described another fetus of similar age as being the length of a finger and having a complete human form, although its bones were still soft.[55] From a modern standpoint, many of these observations are wrong. The difficulty in determining the time of conception that ancient researchers faced continued to be a problem.

The issue of when the fetus was fully formed and thus ready to receive a divinely created soul became less rather than more clear over the course of the sixteenth century. Did being "fully formed" mean that a fetus had all the parts of a human and just got bigger from that point on? Or did it merely mean that the fetus had achieved a humanlike form, in which case development might be seen as a more gradual process and forty-five days a somewhat arbitrary point for ensoulment? Many of the observations of fetuses made by early modern anatomists center on the question of when the fetus is fully formed. Obviously, this was a critical moment in generation because this was when the fetus was supposed to be ensouled by God. Yet depending on which anatomist you read, you could find evidence that a fetus as young as fourteen days was fully formed, or that fetuses did not have human form until at least forty days after conception.

Zerbi's observations that (male) fetuses have human form and the capacity to sense at forty days seems consistent with the traditional Galenic account of reproduction. But his (and Aristotle's) claim that such fetuses are the size of ants is contradicted by Coiter's description of such fetuses as the size of a finger. And while in Bauhin's images the fetuses look like tiny little human beings, Coiter and Zerbi describe creatures that are humanlike but not exactly human. Their proportions are different, certainly from adult humans, but also from babies. And the comparisons of these young fetuses to animals (ants and crabs) suggests a less-than-human state. Further, anatomists like Platter and Coiter who investigated the bones of fetuses and compared them to those of babies, children, and adults became aware of the degree to which skeletal development is incomplete until several years after birth. In sum, certain anatomical observations seemed to support traditional views of fetal development while others called it into question.

Today we can, with a simple Google search, access images and descriptions of every stage of fetal development from fertilization to birth. Yet most of us would balk at attending the dissection of a fetus or newborn. In the past, the dissections of fetuses and young children do not seem to have been transgressive or taboo. One might expect to see some distinction made between a fetus before and after ensoulment, but early modern anatomists dissected fetuses of all ages, as well as stillborn babies and deceased neonates, without any qualms.

Not only were contemporaries not shocked by the activities of anatomists, but a broader public than just physicians and medical students was interested in fetal anatomy. Recall that Colombo witnessed a public dissection of a one-month-old fetus in front of "an assembly of illustrious men and nobles," not just medical men. When the artist Jan van Neck painted the Dutch anatomist Frederik Ruysch, he depicted him in the act of dissecting a newborn (the placenta is still attached) and with a child's skeleton off to one side.[56] Human reproduction fascinated many early modern Europeans, not just physicians. Modern images and descriptions of blastocysts and embryos and fetuses are more accurate than those in early modern anatomy texts. But both premodern and modern sources are alike in depicting the growing fetus as a separate entity, obscuring its connection to and impact on the maternal body.

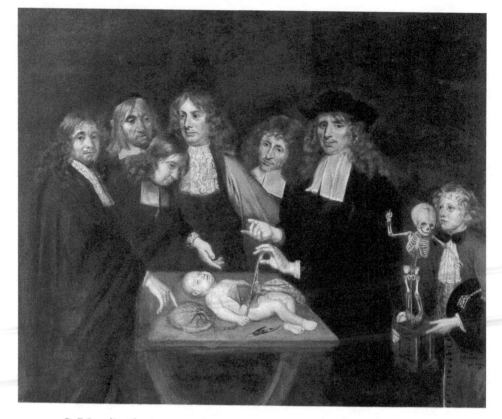

B. F. Landis, *The Anatomy of Dr. Frederik Ruysch*, 1909–1910, after Jan van Neck, 1683. Ruysch lifts the umbilical cord of a dead infant to demonstrate the connection between the infant's body and the placenta. On the far right, Ruysch's son holds one of Ruysch's mounted skeletons of a baby. Wellcome Collection, London.

FETUSES IN JARS

In the seventeenth century, Dutch anatomists developed new methods for preserving anatomical specimens, including fetuses. One of the first to do this was Lodewijk de Bils, who invented a method in which he injected a waxy substance into the veins and arteries of cadavers and then soaked the body in an alcohol solution. He claimed he could stave off decay so that the body could be used for research or anatomy lessons for decades. De Bils's first specimens included "an aborted embryo."[57] But the real rock star of seventeenth- and eighteenth-century anatomical preservation was the anatomist, surgeon, obstetrician, and "medical entrepreneur," Frederik Ruysch (1638–1731).[58] Ruysch developed and perfected a new technique to preserve bodies. Like de Bils, Ruysch injected a mixture of "wax, cinnabar, oil of lavender and coloured pigments" into the veins and arteries and placed the cadaver or body part in a concoction of "nantic brandy and black pepper."[59] Ruysch opened a museum and admitted paying guests to see his anatomical specimens.

Ruysch had a significant interest in fetal specimens, which he obtained from midwives and his own patients when they miscarried or their babies were stillborn.[60] His most famous exhibits were a whole series of "dioramas" in which he posed fetal skeletons among various preserved body parts. He displayed these dioramas in a museum in his house that was open to anyone who could pay the entry fee.[61] But these were just the tip of the iceberg.

Ruysch had numerous miscarried and aborted fetuses, as well as newborns who were either stillborn or died soon after birth, in jars in his collection. Historian Rina Knoeff describes some of the negotiations between Ruysch and the parents of the fetuses and babies in his collection. In one case, Ruysch was called to attend a woman in labor with twins. When the babies did not survive, Ruysch asked the parents for permission to preserve them. In return, he promised them free entrance to his museum so they could visit their babies whenever they wanted. Apparently, the couple did visit. In another case, Ruysch deferred to the parents' wishes that a miscarried embryo be displayed without the attached placenta. Ruysch claimed that many parents expressed gratitude to him for restoring their lost fetuses and infants to a lifelike appearance and preserving them.[62] Visitors from all over Europe flocked to this museum. The Russian

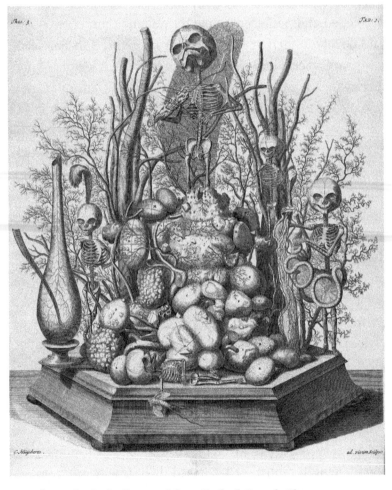

One of Ruysch's fetal "dioramas," from Frederik Ruysch, *Thesaurus anatomicus primus*. Wellcome Collection, London

czar Peter the Great was one of these visitors, and he was so impressed that in 1716 he purchased the collection and moved it to Saint Petersburg.[63] Of the approximately two thousand specimens that the czar purchased, over nine hundred survive, including numerous fetuses.[64]

The preservation techniques developed by Dutch anatomists soon spread all over Europe and subsequently to the United States. Anatomical museums containing preserved cadavers and body parts became de rigueur in medical schools, surgeons' guilds, and scientific societies. And many physicians and surgeons had their own private collections of anatomical specimens. These specimens did not just sit in jars collecting dust while bored medical students filed past them. Rather, specimens were routinely taken out of the jars and handled.[65] By the eighteenth century they were examined with microscopes as well. Preserved specimens were considered essential to research and teaching. Fetal specimens figured prominently in these museums. They were seen as critical to the study of reproduction as well as to the teaching of obstetrics.

In 1836 the Scottish surgeon Frederick Knox (1794–1873) published a manual titled *The Anatomist's Instructor, and Museum Companion: Being Practical Directions for the Formation and Subsequent Management of Anatomical Museums.*[66] As the title suggests, he explained how to prepare anatomical specimens and detailed the type of specimens a well-stocked museum should have. Knox had a great deal of practical experience, having worked at the museum of the Royal College of Surgeons cataloging the collection and preparing new specimens.[67] It was critical to have fetuses of different ages in an anatomical collection because "most circumstances connected with foetal life still require vast elucidation." He noted the difficulty of obtaining enough specimens and opined that while dissection of animal fetuses was useful, it was no substitute for the dissection of human fetuses.[68]

At the University of Leipzig, the chair of anatomy, Wilhelm His (1831–1904), "embarked on a major study of the anatomy of the human embryo" in 1878, a study which required hundreds of fetuses. Rather than preserving the fetuses in jars, His sliced them into very thin sections suitable for examination under a microscope. His especially prized the smallest fetuses, those under two months old. These were exceedingly difficult to obtain. Many women would not even know they were miscarrying this early in pregnancy. And even if they did, what emerged would not look like a fetus. His convinced his wide network of obstetrician colleagues to search carefully through chamber pots of clotted blood in hopes of finding the tiniest embryos. He was able to obtain seventy-nine such "treasures."[69]

American student Franklin Mall (1862–1917) worked with His on the embryo study, becoming familiar with the techniques of sectioning, staining, and preserving embryos and fetuses.[70] When Mall returned to the United States in 1886, he taught anatomy at Clark University and the University of Chicago. And he began amassing an embryo collection of his own. Like His, he contacted obstetricians and asked them to send him "material" from miscarriages and abortions. He included in his requests detailed instructions on how to preserve embryos and fetuses in alcohol for transport.

Many doctors were quite willing to collaborate with Mall and would not have found his requests unusual. Embryo collecting was already happening in the United States before Mall. In the second half of the nineteenth century, American doctors gradually began replacing midwives at the bedsides of laboring

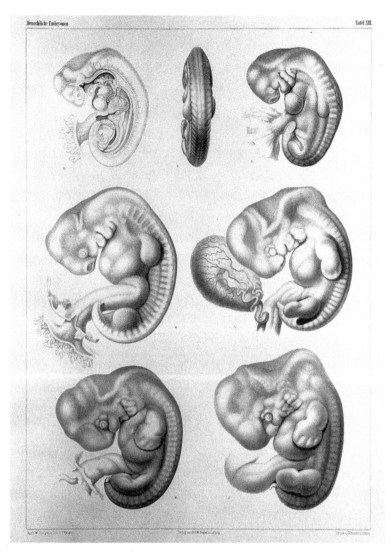

Thinly sliced sections of fetuses, from Wilhelm His, *Anatomie menschlicher Embryonen*. Wellcome Collection, London.

women and were increasingly called in cases of miscarriage as well. "As physicians became more and more involved in the treatment of miscarriage and its complications," writes historian Shannon Withycombe, "they often walked away from such cases with the resulting material products."[71] Since doctors typically cared for women in their homes, taking away miscarried fetuses or stillborn infants required negotiation with the family. Although some parents refused such requests, many agreed. As Withycombe demonstrates in her book *Lost*, few American women in this period experienced miscarriage as the loss of a baby in the way that many American women in the late twentieth and early twenty-first centuries do.[72] However, doctors sometimes resorted to subterfuge to remove desirable fetal specimens from the homes of unwilling patients. In the antebellum South, many doctors obtained fetuses from enslaved women, who of course had no say in the matter. Many, if not most, of the fetal specimens in the museums of southern medical schools and medical societies, as well as the private collections of southern physicians, were the miscarried or stillborn offspring of enslaved women and girls.[73]

When Mall was appointed chair in anatomy at Johns Hopkins University in 1893, he continued his embryo collection project in Baltimore. In 1913, Mall was appointed head of the newly established Department of Embryology at the Carnegie Institute. Like his teacher His, Mall was keen to get very young embryos in his collection to elucidate the early events of embryonic development. Mall assembled a collection of over eight hundred embryos, but the very youngest ones eluded him and other embryologists.

The work of the Carnegie Human Embryo Collection continued after Mall's death. The goal was to have a complete series of specimens of the earliest phases of embryonic development from a fertilized egg to a fourteen-day-old, preimplantation embryo. These "last elusive specimens to round out the Carnegie embryo pantheon," as Lynn Morgan describes them, were donated by a team of researchers in Boston between 1938 and 1954.[74] The team was composed of John Rock (1890–1984), a prominent gynecologist and fertility expert, best known for his role in the development of the birth control pill; Miriam Menkin (1901–92), Rock's lab technician, best known for being the first person to achieve in vitro fertilization of a human egg; and Arthur Hertig (1904–90), a gynecological pathologist. To get very early embryos, the three researchers asked women who were scheduled to have hysterectomies to have unprotected sex in the month prior to the operation. The women had to be married and to have given birth to at least three full-term babies, and they had to be willing to record the dates of their menstrual periods and dates on which they had intercourse. After Rock performed the hysterectomy, Hertig searched the uterus and Fallopian tubes for embryos. Out of 211 operations, he found thirty-four embryos. The earliest was only two cells, estimated to be thirty hours old. The oldest was seventeen days. There is no evidence that any of the researchers, including Rock who was a devout Catholic, or any of the women who participated in the study, had any moral qualms about deliberately creating embryos to be used as specimens.

Most of the fetuses in jars that survive from the eighteenth, nineteenth, and twentieth centuries are no longer on public display, although there are a few exceptions. The Chicago Museum of Science and Industry has an exhibit titled "Your Beginning" containing twenty-four embryos and fetuses that range in age from twenty-eight days to thirty-eight weeks.[75] The collection was assembled in the 1930s by Dr. Helen Button, one of the first female obstetricians at Cook County Hospital, and first displayed at the 1933 Chicago World's Fair.[76] The exhibit is now housed in a "darkened gallery to allow for quiet reflection."[77] As Sara Dubow writes, since these specimens were first shown in the 1930s, there has been a dramatic change in attitudes toward fetuses. In the context of intense debates about abortion beginning in the 1970s, fetuses have shifted from being "curiosities and specimens inspiring wonder and awe into 'babies' and 'human bodies' deserving sympathy and burial."[78] The use of darkened, quiet spaces reflects this new sensibility, carving out a church-like sacred space amid a secular science museum.

Although we may never see actual fetuses, unless we visit exhibits like the one in Chicago, we are surrounded by images of them. Most of the images of fetuses that we see in textbooks, ultrasound screens, pro-life websites, car advertisements, and a million other places show the fetus alone. The classic example of this is the iconic set of photographs titled "A Child Is Born" created by the Swedish photographer Lennart Nilsson in 1965. These images show the stages of human development from conception to birth. The photographs are stunning. Nilsson wanted to see, and to make visible to others, the stages of embryonic and fetal development that took place in the dark and hidden space of the female body. But the maternal body is completely excluded from Nilsson's photographs. His fetuses appear to float against dark backgrounds, like tiny astronauts in a vast universe. In their splendid isolation they resemble their earlier counterparts, the fetuses in jars. Of course, Nilsson had no way of inserting a camera into a living woman's womb to photograph a living fetus. His glorious images of the beginnings of human life are photographs of dead fetuses. One is reminded of the artistry of Frederik Ruysch, making dead fetuses appear lifelike. In a widely cited article, Rosalind Petchesky argued that the prevalence of such images, even when they do not appear in explicitly pro-life contexts, encourages us to see the fetus "as primary and autonomous, the woman as absent or peripheral."[79] But this view of the fetus long predates the use of modern image-making technologies. It has been central to the study of human reproduction since antiquity.

MATERNAL MORBIDITY AND MORTALITY

The implications of seeing the fetus as "primary and autonomous" and the pregnant person as "absent or peripheral" extend beyond the abortion debate. The combination of thinking of fetuses as babies and thinking about fetal development as separate from pregnancy has had disastrous implications for the health of both mothers and babies. As the pro-life movement in this country has gained strength, rates of maternal mortality and morbidity in the United States have risen, until we now have the highest rates of any wealthy country. The new fixation on the fetus as a person and a patient has exacerbated the old tendency to neglect the pregnant person. There is, of course, no one simple explanation for the alarming rise in maternal mortality and morbidity, but it is consistent with a long history of downplaying the significance of the female body to fetal development.

One manifestation of this is the high maternal mortality numbers in the United States. We have the dubious distinction of having a higher maternal mortality rate than any other wealthy, industrialized country. Maternal mortality includes not just deaths during pregnancy or childbirth; it includes deaths up to forty-two days after the end of the pregnancy "from any cause related to or aggravated by the pregnancy or its management."[80] In 2018, there were 17.4 maternal deaths for every 100,000 live births in the United States. For comparison, in France, which has the next highest rate, there were 8.7 maternal deaths for every 100,000 live births. In New Zealand and Norway, which have the lowest ratios, there were fewer than 2.0 maternal deaths per 100,000 live births.[81] Further, although there has been a worldwide reduction in maternal mortality over the past twenty-five years, maternal mortality rates in the United States have been rising since the 1990s.[82]

Repeatedly, studies have shown that most maternal deaths are preventable.[83] For example, preeclampsia accounts for 8 percent of maternal deaths in the United States. This is a complication of pregnancy characterized by high blood pressure. Left untreated, it can lead to kidney or liver damage and death. Preeclampsia can appear during pregnancy, but also in the weeks after birth. Even so, many obstetricians are not trained to recognize the signs of preeclampsia, especially when they occur after the birth. Although neonates are monitored very closely in hospitals, postpartum women often are not. Preeclampsia deaths are eminently preventable. In Britain, where the diagnosis and treatment of preeclampsia are standardized and medical personnel are trained in how to recognize and treat the condition, there were two preeclampsia deaths between 2012 and 2014. In the United States, fifty to seventy women die of preeclampsia each year.[84]

"Where Is the "M" in Maternal-Fetal Medicine?" Dr. Mary D'Alton, professor and chair of the Department of Obstetrics and Gynecology at Columbia and a specialist in maternal fetal medicine, posed this question in a commentary in the journal *Ob-*

stetrics and Gynecology in 2010. D'Alton called for greater attention to the health of pregnant and postpartum women and pointed out that the field of maternal-fetal medicine developed in the 1970s as a subspecialty of obstetrics focused on high-risk pregnancies. The field has made substantial clinical advances in the last four decades, but these have almost all been in the care of fetuses and newborns. Maternal-fetal specialists, in D'Alton's view, are far better trained and equipped to deal with fetuses than with pregnant women. For example, she notes that in recent years there has been a decrease in the use of forceps in deliveries and in breech vaginal deliveries. Instead, the rate of Caesarean sections has risen, and Caesareans carry a higher risk of death or injury than vaginal births. Yet very few maternal-fetal specialists are trained in these lower-risk delivery options.[85] Since D'Alton's first call to action, the Society for Maternal-Fetal Medicine has spearheaded an effort to improve maternal care, but more needs to be done.[86]

Maternal mortality is a critical measure of health, and accounts of new mothers dying hours or days after giving birth are heartrending, but another serious problem is maternal morbidity, that is, rates of maternal health problems in the weeks and months after birth. Even the healthiest, least complicated pregnancies entail physical changes that go well beyond morning sickness, enlarged breasts, and an expanding abdomen. These changes can last long after birth, and some can be permanent.

Further, pregnancy complications, some of them life-threatening, are far more common than most people believe. A study published in 1994 reported that in the United States, around 22 percent of pregnant people experienced complications severe enough to require hospitalization.[87] Data from the

Centers for Disease Control and Prevention (CDC) shows that pregnancy complications increased between 1993 and 2014.[88] Maternal morbidity has attracted less attention than mortality, but also considerably less attention than fetal and infant health. One study cited by D'Alton reported that "severe maternal morbidity—defined as peripartum transfusion, hysterectomy, or eclampsia—was 50 times more common than maternal death," and another "found that 31% of patients, the equivalent of 1.2 million women, experienced some type of morbidity during their delivery hospitalization." Maternal morbidity includes many conditions that are not life-threatening but can seriously compromise quality of life, such as fatigue, pain, sleep disorders, pain during intercourse, and depression.[89]

Although we ought to care about the health of new parents because their well-being matters, it is also the case that the health of mothers influences the health of children. Studies have found that "poor maternal physical health was related to children's reduced general physical health, frequent tantrums, and difficulty in playing with other children, as well as mothers' feeling of difficulties in managing children's behaviors at 3 years of age."[90] Postpartum care in the United States is generally limited to one doctor's visit six weeks after giving birth, during which a woman gets a vaginal exam and advice on contraception. Surveys consistently show that many women find this inadequate to address the full range of problems they experience after birth. As one woman described her experience, "I was just a vessel for the baby, and my health was important only up until I was no longer the vessel."[91] Calls for reform include extending routine postpartum care a full year and providing home health care. In many other countries, nurses or other health care professionals visit new mothers at home. Compounding these issues, the

United States is one of the very few countries in the world that has no paid leave for parents following birth.[92]

Maternal mortality and morbidity are exponentially higher among Black women. Compared to white women, African American women are at least three times as likely to die from complications arising from pregnancy or labor.[93] Black women have higher rates of C-sections, postoperative complications to C-sections, preeclampsia, peripartum cardiomyopathy, and post-partum depression.[94] This makes the lack of adequate postpar-tum care a much bigger risk for Black women. Further, racial biases among medical professionals compromise the care of Black women. In interviews with over two hundred Black mothers conducted by reporters for ProPublica and NPR in 2017, "the feeling of being devalued and disrespected by medical pro-viders was a constant theme." "Black expectant and new mothers frequently told us that doctors and nurses didn't take their pain seriously," report Martin and Montague.[95] This is con-sistent with studies that show doctors do not take Black people's pain seriously.[96] It is also consistent with a long history of ne-glecting maternal health and well-being.

We may have advanced beyond Aristotle and Hippocrates in many respects, but we still view the pregnant body as a mere vessel in which the fetus is formed, the oven in which the bun is baked. And if we think the maternal body is not doing much besides incubating the developing baby, we do not have much incentive to devote resources to maternal health and well-being. Medical advice for pregnant women has long concentrated on the lifestyle choices—diet, exercise, and rest—thought to be healthiest for the fetus. For example, the CDC recommends that all pregnant women and women who could potentially become pregnant consume at least four hundred micrograms of folic acid a day.[97] This advice emerges from the centuries-long history of studying the intricacies of fetal development. Folic acid is essential to the formation of the fetus's neural tube, and low levels of folic acid in the mother's diet raise the risk of birth defects, including spina bifida and anencephaly. While this advice is sound, folic acid consumption is intended to support the development of the fetus, not the health of the mother.

Improving maternal health—and addressing the racial inequalities in maternal health—will take more than vitamins. It requires a holistic approach to the myriad social and economic factors that impact maternal well-being. Monica Casper points out that many of the most pro-life states, the ones where abortion is now severely restricted or outright banned, are the same ones that refused to accept Medicaid expansion in 2020. And yet, multiple studies show that Medicaid expansion significantly decreases infant and maternal mortality. "One of the benefits to infants of increasing access to care," writes Casper, "is healthier pregnant women."[98] A 2021 report by the Commonwealth Fund on "Policies for Reducing Maternal Morbidity and Mortality and Enhancing Equity in Maternal Health" advised ensuring that pregnant and potentially pregnant people have access to safe housing and neighborhoods, healthy food, education, and employment.[99]

Addressing what are known as the "social determinants of health" will have more impact on rates of maternal morbidity and mortality than any medical advances in obstetrical care. Expanding Medicaid and tackling the social determinants of health are not policies that emerge from the study of fetal development. Rather, they emerge from an understanding of fetuses as inextricably linked to the bodies and to the lives of the people who gestate them.

CONCLUSION

The first (and only) time I encountered fetuses in jars was the year after I graduated from college. I worked as a lab technician in a reproductive biology lab in Philadelphia. I attended, with other members of the lab, a conference held at the Mütter Museum, a medical museum established in the nineteenth century by the College of Physicians of Philadelphia. At a break in the conference, I took the opportunity to tour the museum. There was a temporary exhibit on obstetrics, which had forceps and other instruments from the eighteenth and nineteenth centuries, as well as a large collection of fetuses in jars, many of them with gross abnormalities. It was painful to look at. The forceps looked disturbingly like torture instruments, and I could not stop thinking about the agonizing deaths many of the women who had once carried these fetuses must have suffered.

I was guided around this exhibit by a male medical student. He clearly did not share my discomfort and enthusiastically drew my attention to specimen after specimen. Being young and impressionable, I decided I needed to cultivate greater objectivity as well as more appreciation for the heroes of modern obstetrics. Then we came to one tiny specimen in the corner of the exhibit, the only one derived from a male body, testicles deformed by illness or accident. At this point my guide's eyes widened in horror, and he turned rapidly away saying, "I can't look at that!" So different was his response to the testicles than to the fetuses and forceps that I at first thought he was making a self-deprecating joke. He was, however, entirely serious. Noting that clinical detachment had its limits, I took my time examining the testicles and then trailed after him.

When I look back on this encounter, I see two different views of history. I saw each of the fetuses suspended in formaldehyde as a fragment of a personal history, the sole remaining relic of the life story of a long-dead woman. He saw them as part of a different history, the history of how we came to know about the normal and abnormal course of embryonic development. Neither narrative is wrong, and both are important. But they have been kept separate for so long that we no longer see how intertwined they are.

3

THE DANGEROUS WOMB

In January 2020, Brittney Poolaw, a twenty-year-old Oklahoma woman, miscarried. She was between fifteen and seventeen weeks pregnant. When she went to the hospital, she was asked about drug use, and she admitted to using marijuana and methamphetamine. Hospital personnel contacted the police, and Poolaw was arrested and charged with manslaughter. Unable to pay the $20,000 bail, Poolaw spent eighteen months in jail until her case finally went to trial in October 2021. The medical examiner testified that while Poolaw's fetus had tested positive for methamphetamine, there was no conclusive evidence that Poolaw's drug use had been a factor in her miscarriage. The autopsy of Poolaw's fetus had also "detected a congenital abnormality, placental abruption and chorioamnionitis," all of which were more likely causes of miscarriage than methamphetamine use. Despite this testimony, a jury found Poolaw guilty.[1]

In recent years there has been a marked increase in prosecutions of women who miscarry. The first American woman to be convicted of "feticide" was Purvi Patel of Indiana. In 2013 Patel went into premature labor when she was twenty-three or twenty-four weeks pregnant. The baby died shortly after birth. There was no evidence that Patel did anything to induce labor early or to harm her baby once it was born. Nonetheless, she was convicted and sentenced to twenty years in prison, a conviction that was overturned in 2016.[2] Women who face criminal prosecution for miscarriage are almost all poor, and they are disproportionately women of color. Poolaw, a member of the Wichita and Affiliated Tribes, fits this pattern.

These cases illuminate a deep continuity in the history of medicine, namely, the idea that wombs—and women's bodies generally—are dangerous places. From the earliest medical writings in ancient Greece, doctors did not imagine the womb as a warm, safe, and comfortable home. Rather, they believed the fetus was from the moment of conception imprisoned in a hostile environment. To understand the current tendency to control and punish pregnant women, and to blame them for poor birth outcomes, we need to understand this tradition, because it continues to underlie a great deal of the medical understanding of pregnancy and fetal development.

The notion that the womb is a dangerous place for a fetus will seem profoundly counterintuitive. Until extremely recently, the only place conception could occur was in a woman's uterus. The first successful human in vitro fertilization that resulted in a baby took place in 1978. Even now, the failure rate of IVF is high. Although scientists can coax sperm to fertilize eggs in a laboratory, the resulting embryos cannot develop into fetuses outside the womb. Before the mid-twentieth century, a fetus that left the womb too early could not survive. And although neonatal care for premature infants has improved dramatically, standard medical procedure in cases where premature birth is feared is to attempt to delay labor. In sum, even in our high-tech world, women's bodies are essential to the production of babies. Science fiction fantasies aside, this will be true for the foreseeable future. Why then is there such concern about the safety and security of the fetus in the womb?

BLOOD AND POISON

Fears about the dangers of the womb are expressed in some of the earliest medical texts. From the time of Aristotle (384–322 BCE) and Hippocrates (c. 460–c. 377 BCE) in ancient Greece, medical and philosophical writers accepted that fetuses were nourished in the womb by their mothers' blood. However, this blood was frequently equated with menstrual blood, which many Greeks believed was toxic. This lent a peculiar ambivalence to the pregnant body, because it both nourished and poisoned.

This requires some explanation of Greek views of menstruation and menstrual blood. Menstruation was not connected to the female reproductive cycle of periodic ovulation until the nineteenth century. Until that time, menstrual blood was understood as a waste product analogous to urine or feces. Just as these latter substances were the residual products of digestion, so too was menstrual blood. Menstrual blood accumulated in the uterus in the same way that urine accumulated in the bladder and feces accumulated in the large intestine. And just as the bladder and colon required regular evacuation to remove the accumulated wastes, so too did the uterus.

The fact that women menstruate and men do not, was, for the Greeks, a mark of the superiority of the male body. The male body was hot and dry, where the female body was cold and wet.

This did not mean that male body temperature was noticeably higher. Rather, it meant that men had more life force, more vitality. Male bodies were harder, with more sinew and muscle, corresponding to the more active, aggressive, and rational quality of the male psyche. Women's bodies, by contrast, were softer and weaker, corresponding to the passive, submissive, and irrational female character.[3] The hotter, drier male body consumed food more thoroughly and efficiently than the colder, wetter female body, which meant that women's bodies produced more waste residue and needed an extra mode of evacuation. This was why women menstruated and men did not. During pregnancy and lactation, the excess food that would have been excreted as menstrual blood was used to feed the baby, first as blood in the womb and then as milk in the breasts. For over two thousand years, the uterus was an organ with a dual function. It was both a repository for waste products and the place where new life was generated.[4] Menstrual blood, too, had a dual character. It was waste product, and as such, toxic and dangerous. But it was also food for the growing fetus.

Ambivalence about menstrual blood comes through in discussions of conception and fetal development. Aristotle wrote that menstrual blood in women was analogous to semen in men.[5] But whereas semen was active, menstrual blood was passive. Semen provided the active principle, the life force, the soul of the offspring. Menstrual blood was just the material out of which the embryo was formed. Aristotle wrote: "The contribution which the female makes to generation is the *matter* used therein, [and] that this is to be found in the substance constituting the menstrual fluid."[6] The analogy that Aristotle used was that semen was an artisan, the living, dynamic force crafting an object. Menstrual blood was the material used by that artisan. Menstrual blood was the wood the carpenter used to build the house, or the clay the potter used to shape a vessel.[7] Menstrual blood was necessary, but it played a subordinate role in generation to semen.

But more than just passive and subordinate, menstrual blood was dirty and disgusting in a way that semen was not. Aristotle wrote that "the female . . . lacks the power to concoct semen out of the final state of the nourishment . . . because of the coldness of its nature." He adds, "Just as lack of concoction produces in the bowels diarrhoea, so in the blood-vessels it produces discharges of blood of various sorts, and especially the menstrual discharge." Although he notes that menstrual blood is a "natural discharge" and diarrhea is a "morbid" discharge,[8] his comparison highlights the dual nature of menstrual blood. It is certainly necessary to reproduction, but it is like feces, urine, and diarrhea in a way that semen, which is also a "concoction" of food, is not. Semen is refined; menstrual blood is always somewhat tainted and impure.

At least two texts in the Hippocratic Corpus describe conception, pregnancy, and birth: *Generation* and *On the Nature of the Child*. The author of *Generation*, like Aristotle, asserts that semen and menses are analogous, evidenced by the fact that girls begin menstruating at about the same age that boys begin producing semen.[9] The author of *On the Nature of the Child* explains that when a woman is pregnant, she ceases to menstruate. The blood that would have accumulated in the uterus and been expelled every month is drawn to the developing fetus.[10] This text also equates menstrual blood, normally a waste product, and the blood that nourishes a developing fetus, allowing it to grow to full size. The author expounds on the toxic nature of menstrual blood when he discusses problems faced by women who are not pregnant but fail to menstruate. The uterus becomes excessively hot from the retained menstrual blood and can spread this heat to other parts of the body. This can cause "swellings," and "there is sometimes a danger that a woman will be actually crippled when this happens." The engrossed uterus presses on the bladder and blocks the passage of urine, or it presses against "the hip or the lumbar regions, causing pain there."[11] Trapped in the body, menstrual blood is a dangerous substance. Women are at their most fertile right after menstruation has stopped: "It is when the womb and veins are empty that women conceive; hence the most favorable time for conception is just after menstruation."[12] A cleansed womb, one free of menstrual blood, was the most suitable environment for conception to occur. At other times of the month, when the womb is partially full of menstrual blood, the chances of conception were diminished, although not eliminated. The Hippocratic writers, like Aristotle, saw menstrual blood both as food for the fetus and as something filthy and dangerous.[13]

The ancient Roman physician Soranus of Ephesus (second century CE) also asserted that the best time to try to conceive a baby was "when menstruation is ending and abating" because at that time the uterus was cleansed of menstrual blood and ready to receive semen.[14] Failure to menstruate was dangerous because it meant menstrual blood was trapped in the body. Retention of menses might cause "heaviness of the head, dimness of vision, pain in the joints, sensitiveness at the base of the eyes, of the loins and the lower abdomen, discomfort, tossing about, upset stomach, and sometimes chills and fever."[15] But menstrual blood was also nourishment, essential to the formation and growth of the fetus and infant.

The capacity of menstrual blood to both nourish and poison was affirmed by medieval medical and scientific writers.[16] One text stated that "every human being . . . is generated from the seed of the father and the menses of the mother."[17] But the same text included the assertion that "women are so full of venom in the time of their menstruation that they poison animals by their glance; they infect children in the cradle; they spot the cleanest mirror; and whenever men have sexual intercourse with them they are made leprous and sometimes cancerous."[18] The notions that menstruating women could cause wine to sour, milk to curdle, and mirrors to become cloudy were integral to both popular and scientific understandings of women's bodies.[19] Menstruating women were sometimes compared to basilisks, semi-mythical snakelike creatures that were so poisonous they could kill a person or animal just by looking at them or breathing on them. Like the glance of a menstruating woman, the basilisk's gaze exuded a powerful and deadly venom. The alchemical text *On the Nature of Things*, attributed (probably incorrectly) to sixteenth-century alchemist Paracelsus, made this connection startlingly concrete. The author informs readers that it is possible to create a basilisk by taking a man's sperm and placing it in a vessel with menstrual blood. If you incubate the vessel at a constant warm temperature for an unspecified time, a basilisk will emerge.[20] This was uncomfortably close to the way babies were thought to be generated: by placing the man's sperm into the "vessel" of the woman's uterus and nourishing it with menstrual blood.

SMALLPOX

In the Middle Ages, the dangers of menstrual blood to the developing fetus were most extensively elaborated in an unexpected place: medical writing on smallpox. Smallpox was first identified as a distinct disease, separate from the more generic category of "fevers," by the ninth-century Persian physician Abu Bakr Muhammad ibn Zakariya al Razi, known in Europe as Rhazes (c. 850–925).[21] By this time, smallpox was an endemic disease throughout the Middle East, Europe, Asia, and parts of Africa. It was widely recognized that once a person had smallpox, they did not get it again. It was also widely recognized that a very high percentage of young children suffered from the disease. The majority survived and never had smallpox again; a minority succumbed to the disease. In the tenth century, another Persian physician, 'Ali ibn al-'Abbas al-Majusi (died 982–994 CE), known in Europe as Haly Abbas, came up with what would become the dominant explanation for all this.

Haly Abbas accounted for the high prevalence of smallpox in children (and the rarity of the disease in adults) by asserting that smallpox was caused by menstrual blood. All children, he noted, were nourished in their mothers' wombs with menstrual blood. Some of this blood was left in the child's body after it was born. Menstrual blood was a toxic substance, so this was an unstable situation. Sometime in the first few years of life, the child's body would attempt to purge itself of the remnants of menstrual blood still remaining in the blood. Haly Abbas interpreted the symptoms of smallpox, which included fevers, pain, rashes, and pustules, as the body's efforts to purge residual menstrual toxins from the body. Most children survived this purging and emerged healthier, with purified blood, but some were overcome by the poison. The very rare cases of adults with smallpox were explained by the failure of their bodies to expel the menstrual blood when they were children, forcing this process to occur later in life than it should. This was a perfectly logical explanation of the observed clinical picture of smallpox, but it was a logic that reflected highly misogynistic assumptions inherited from ancient Greek physicians about the impurity of the female body.

A century later, the Persian physician Ibn-Sīnā (c. 980–1037), known in Europe as Avicenna, incorporated Haly Abbas's ideas about smallpox into his monumental *Canon of Medicine*.[22] The *Canon* was translated into Latin in the twelfth century by Gerard of Cremona (c. 1114–1187) and became the most important medical text in Europe, used in European medical schools until the seventeenth century.[23] Thus "canonized," Haly Abbas's explanation of smallpox became the dominant explanation of this very common disease in the Arabic-speaking world and, later, in Latin translation, in Europe.

In the Middle Ages, the European understanding of smallpox was basically taken over wholesale from Haly Abbas and Avicenna. Europeans saw it as a disease of children and as an almost inevitable part of growing up. This is reflected in medical writing for the next five centuries from physicians across Europe. In the early thirteenth century, the physician Gilbert the Englishman (1180–1250) wrote that "smallpox is caused when a child is conceived during the mother's menstrual period or if the nourishment it receives in the womb has not been purified of menstrual blood."[24] The thirteenth-century French doctor and medical professor Bernard de Gordon (fl. 1270–1330) claimed that smallpox was "generated from menstrual blood retained in the porosities of the fetal parts."[25] The thirteenth-century English physician John of Gaddesden (c. 1280–1361) wrote that smallpox "came from the corruption of the menstrual blood."[26] The fourteenth-century Portuguese physician Valesco de Tarenta (fl. 1382–1418) wrote that smallpox and measles (the two diseases were often linked) were caused by menstrual blood that insinuated itself into the body of the developing fetus. "The fetus is nourished by the purer part" of the mother's blood, he asserted, "but the filthy parts are retained in the porosities."[27] All of these men wrote texts that were read and cited for several centuries.

Although the idea of menstrual contamination causing smallpox was criticized in the sixteenth and seventeenth centuries, it retained a place as a valid opinion. At the end of the sixteenth century, Simon Kellwaye noted that physicians disagreed about the cause of smallpox, but one prominent explanation was still the "menstruall bloud which from the beginning in our Mothers wombes wee receaved."[28] In his account of smallpox, the Dutch physician Isbrand van Diemerbroeck (1609–1674) noted that there were "various and great Contentions among the most Eminent Physitians" over the causes of smallpox. One of these explanations was still "the Impurity of the Mothers Blood" and the "Defilement" that had to be purged from the body after birth.[29] And some medical writers, like Anthony Westwood, continued to regard menstrual contamination as the sole correct explanation for smallpox:

> That the mothers blood is the true cause of the Small Pox and Measles, and that is hence chiefly gathered, because among many thousands of men it is hard to find one, who once in his life hath not had these diseases. . . . It remains therefore that the Small Pox and Measles spring from the Mothers Blood, with which the child is nourished in the womb; for therein, be it never so pure, some impurities are found, which communicate their pollution to the parts

of the child; and that pollution of the parts doth defile the masse of blood...."[30]

From the tenth century to the seventeenth, a chorus of medical writers blamed smallpox on mothers. They described menstrual blood as impure, putrid, and corrupt, and they compared it to filth, dregs, pollution, and defilement. For at least five hundred years, medical opinion in the Middle East and Europe held that all mothers poisoned the fetuses they carried. Part of growing up was overcoming this maternal taint.

MATERNAL IMAGINATION

Another medical doctrine that was virtually unquestioned until the nineteenth century was the notion of maternal imagination. The notion that mothers' minds had the power to shape their fetuses in utero is ancient. One of the oldest descriptions is in the Bible.[31] Jacob convinces his father-in-law Laban to give him all the striped, speckled, and spotted cows, sheep, and goats of his flock. And then he cleverly arranges to increase their number. He takes tree branches and peels off strips and flecks of the bark so the branches have white stripes and spots. He then places the striped and spotted branches in front of the watering troughs, where the animals will see them when they come to drink and mate. The animals that conceived while looking at the striped and spotted branches bore young that had stripes and spots, thus increasing Jacob's flock at the expense of Laban's.

The ancient Greeks, too, appear to have given credence to the notion of maternal imagination. The pre-Socratic philosopher Empedocles (fifth century BCE) reportedly said, "Fetuses are shaped by what the woman visualizes around the time of the conception. For often women have fallen in love with statues and paintings and have produced offspring which resemble them."[32] And the physician Soranus noted that "some women, seeing monkeys during intercourse, have borne children resembling monkeys." Like Jacob, Soranus suggested that maternal imagination could be harnessed to good effect. He relates, "The tyrant of the Cyprians who was misshapen, compelled his wife to look at beautiful statues during intercourse and became the father of well-shaped children."[33]

By the sixteenth century, it was widely accepted that anything that made a strong impression on a pregnant woman, especially if it was frightening or repulsive, might leave an imprint on the fetus. All kinds of birthmarks and abnormalities were blamed on maternal imagination. Babies were born with "hare-lips," for example, because their mothers had been startled by rabbits while they were pregnant. So widespread was this belief that many towns and cities forbade butchers to hang rabbits in their windows for fear of their effect on pregnant women.[34]

Both popular and medical literature abounded with stories of babies born deformed in various ways because of maternal imagination. The French surgeon Ambroise Paré (1510–1590) described several cases of "Monsters that are created through the imagination" in his book *On Monsters and Marvels*. These cases included a girl born with hair all over her body because, while having sex, her mother had looked at a picture of John the Baptist dressed in animal pelts; the baby that looked like a frog because his mother had been holding a frog in her hand (a cure for fever) while having sex; or the white princess who gave birth to a Black baby because she looked at a picture of a "Moor" when the baby was conceived.[35]

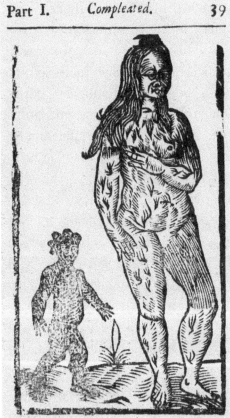

Part I.   *Compleated.*   39

The Effigie of a Maid all Hairy, and an Infan that was Born Black, by the Imagination of their Parents:

The Black baby born to the white princess and the hairy woman, both products of maternal imagination, from *Aristotle's master-piece compleated* (London, 1702), 39. National Library of Medicine, Bethesda, MD.

According to historian Karen Weingarten, the authors of popular health guides in the United States continued to invoke maternal imagination as a cause of congenital anomalies and disabilities until the end of the nineteenth century.[36] Weingarten discusses several of these guides, including Seth Pancoast's *The Ladies' Medical Guide*, first published in 1859, and George H. Napheys's *The Physical Life of Woman: Advice to the Maiden, Wife, and Mother*, first published in 1869. Both books went through numerous editions and reached hundreds of thousands of readers. Pancoast and Napheys insisted that maternal imagination was a scientific fact, validated by centuries of evidence. Both authors cited the biblical story of Jacob increasing his flock by causing the birth of more spotted animals. Both repeated the story about the tyrant who made his wife look at beautiful statues so their children would be beautiful. And Napheys included Paré's story of the white princess who had a Black baby.

In addition to these historical examples, each provided a list of more recent cases. Their examples included women who saw beggars who were missing a hand, or fingers or part of an arm or leg, and then had babies who were missing the corresponding part, women who were startled by mice and lizards and had babies with marks on their bodies in the shape of those animals, a woman who saw a person with a harelip and had a baby with a harelip, a woman who saw someone having an epileptic seizure whose baby was then epileptic, a woman bitten by a dog whose baby was born with bite marks in the same part of his body on which his mother was bitten. Both Pancoast and Napheys asserted that the state of mind and body of both parents at the moment of conception had a powerful influence on the baby. Pancoast stated that "children conceived during or after drunkenness or debauchery, are liable not only to a predisposition to intemperance, but to a debility, both of mind and body, amounting in many instances to idiotcy [sic] itself."[37] Napheys warned that children conceived while the parents were drunk would be epileptic and that the mother's "anger and irritability" would mark the baby.[38]

Sometimes the power of maternal imagination could be harnessed for the benefit of the developing fetus. In Renaissance

Italy, well-to-do brides were given domestic objects like trays and dishes painted with images of the Madonna and Child or the Holy Family.[39] Michelangelo himself painted one of these.[40] The idea was that contemplation of the fat, healthy baby Jesus would encourage the production of fat, healthy male heirs. Doctors advised husbands to treat pregnant wives gently, to avoid upsetting them, and to indulge their cravings for strange foods. Pancoast recommended that pregnant women have "agreeable society, suitable amusements, recreations, and exercise."[41] And Napheys advised: "During pregnancy the mother should often have some painting or engraving representing cheerful and beautiful figures before her eyes, or often contemplate some graceful statue."[42] But even these positive practices suggest a lurking fear of the harm that the mother's imagination could do without proper disciplining. Women, naturally irrational, unstable, and emotional, made poor caretakers of fetuses.

In describing these long-discredited theories of maternal influence on fetal development, my point is not to set up a comforting opposition between then and now, between the superstitions and errors of the past and the science and rationality of the present. Of course, we know that menstrual blood does not cause smallpox. Nor does it cloud mirrors, turn men into lepers, or generate basilisks. We know that women cannot make their babies more beautiful by staring at images of beautiful people, and that being startled by a rabbit, mouse, frog, lizard, or any other creature while pregnant will have no effect on the baby. But we—and here I mean both the medical establishment and the general public—still believe that the major threats to the health and well-being of fetuses come from their own mothers. We have taken old anxieties and clothed them in new scientific garb.

DISCIPLINING THE PREGNANT BODY

The deep-seated fear of the harm the maternal body can do to the fetus has shaped medical understandings of pregnancy and fetal development for centuries. Indeed, this belief continues to inform attitudes toward pregnant women in the present. It would be very hard to find a pregnant woman in America today who has not received unsolicited advice from total strangers about what she should or should not eat, drink, or do because it could hurt her baby. A great deal of the medical and popular advice given to pregnant women over the past two millennia reflects a concern to protect the fetus from its mother. Some of this advice is couched as actions that a pregnant woman can take to create optimal conditions for fetal growth and development. But a great deal of it is warnings about things women should not do because they will damage or kill the fetus.

Attempts to protect fetuses by controlling the diet and behavior of pregnant women have an ancient pedigree. In the second century CE, the Roman physician Soranus gave advice on what a woman should eat and drink during pregnancy, what kind of exercise she should take, and what activities she should avoid. Soranus divided pregnancy into three stages. The first starts at conception and lasts about forty days. The greatest concern in this period is miscarriage, because in these early days the "seed" is easily dislodged and expelled from the uterus. In the first couple of days after conception, the woman should lie "quietly in bed." She should not bathe, and she should try to avoid any strong emotions or mental upset, as well as coughing, sneezing, or vomiting. For the remainder of this first period of pregnancy, she should take only light exercise and should not have sex. She must also take great care of her diet in these early days, both to body a safer, healthier place for her fetus. Foods that are hard to digest decompose in the body, and the fetus is exposed to this rotting, putrid matter rather than pure, nutritious food. This is most apparent in Soranus's recommendations for how to manage women who crave strange or harmful substances like dirt, charcoal, or unripe fruit while pregnant. "One must oppose the desires of pregnant women for harmful things first by arguing that the damage from the things which satisfy the desires in an unreasonable way harms the fetus just as it harms the stomach; because the fetus obtains food which is neither clean nor suitable, but only such food as a body in bad condition can supply."[46]

The last stage of pregnancy is from the seventh month until birth. The primary focus is preparing the woman for birth. At the beginning of this period, she should "partake of more plentiful food" which will increase both her strength as well as that of her fetus.[47] As labor draws near, she should eat less, exercise less, and refrain entirely from sex. The critical importance of following all these rules is underscored in the section on "How to Recognize the Newborn That Is Worth Rearing," where Soranus offers criteria for deciding whether it is worthwhile to offer a newborn care or better to simply let it die. The first thing he says is, "The infant which is suited by nature for rearing will be distinguished by the fact that its mother has spent the period of pregnancy in good health."[48] Break the rules, and even if born alive and in apparent good health, your baby may be deemed unfit.

Over the centuries, the advice to pregnant women on what they should and should not eat and the activities they should and should not engage in have changed with changing medical fashions. But the dire warnings of what can happen if a woman disobeys the rules laid out by medical authorities have not. The tenth-century Persian physician Avicenna wrote that pregnant women needed to avoid "excessive motion" for fear of shaking the fetus loose from the womb and causing a miscarriage. Pregnant women should never engage in vigorous physical activity; they should bathe only infrequently; and they should not have sex. Any of these activities could cause a miscarriage. Avicenna's advice on the best diet to ensure fetal health and well-being included bread made with refined flour instead of whole grains, porridge, lamb stew, and fruits like quinces, apples, pears, and pomegranates.[49] These foods were easily digestible and nutritious. Of course, he listed foods to avoid as well: capers, olives, kidney beans, chickpeas, and sesame.

In the fifteenth century Michele Savonarola (c. 1385–1468), court physician to Niccolò III d'Este, wrote a book about pregnancy dedicated to the women of Ferrara. "If you desire to have a beautiful child, of good complexion and gifted by nature," he wrote, "use good, recommended and easy to digest foods as those listed below."[50] Savonarola advised pregnant women to eat bread made from wheat rather than bread made from coarser grains like bran and to drink light red wine rather than water. Savonarola believed that women could influence the sex of their child by the foods they ate while pregnant. He assured them that if they followed his diet recommendations their baby would be not only healthy but male, a clear priority for many noble families. He also issued dire warnings about the damage women could do to their unborn children if they ate too much or ate the wrong kinds of food. "You should not risk because of the vituperous sin of gluttony loosing or staining such an excellent and worthy fruit through miscarriage," he wrote. He particularly warned women away from fish, fresh fruit, and cold water.[51]

In 1915 Mary M. West wrote a booklet titled *Prenatal Care* for the Children's Bureau of the US Department of Labor. She declared that for pregnant women, "An ideal diet includes a relatively large proportion of liquids, a small proportion of meats, and a correspondingly generous proportion of fresh fruits and vegetables."[52] A pregnant woman should consume "four to eight" glasses of water every day and eat a wide variety of raw or lightly cooked fruits and vegetables. She should also drink milk, cultivating a taste for it if she has not been in the habit of drinking it. Pregnant women should bathe daily but avoid both hot and cold baths. West advised light exercise like leisurely walking and gardening. She was particularly adamant that pregnant women get fresh air. They should sleep with the windows open in all seasons, even sleep outside if possible. In addition, they should spend "at least two hours of each day in the open air, and as much more as possible."[53]

A recurrent theme in pregnancy advice through the centuries is that it is essential for pregnant women to sacrifice their own personal comfort and subordinate their own desires for the good of their fetus. Don't eat too much, says Savonarola, or you will miscarry. Don't like milk? Develop a taste for it, says West. A particularly alarming example of this theme can be found in a syndicated health column written by Dr. William A. Evans, a prominent physician and public health leader in the first half of the twentieth century.[54] Evans wrote a regular column for the *Chicago Tribune* called "How to Keep Well" in which he answered readers' questions. On November 11, 1928, he published an abridged version of a letter sent to him by a "Mrs. E." Mrs. E. offered her experiences as a cautionary tale and asked Evans to publish her story in the "hope [that] this letter will teach many prospective mothers to have maternity care and to obey the rules given them by the doctors." Mrs. E. wrote:

after birth. In the 1920s, infants with Down syndrome were frequently denied medical care and often died young. There is no sense in Evans's paraphrase of Mrs. E.'s letter that the death of a disabled child was a tragedy. Rather, the fact that the baby was not normal and healthy—like his "prize winner" brother—is the tragedy, and it is a tragedy that could have been prevented had Mrs. E. only listened to her doctor's advice. While it is true that the genetic basis of Down syndrome (the nondisjunction of chromosome 21) was not known in 1928, there was no good reason to suspect that it was caused by poor maternal diet. And yet Evans had no compunction about suggesting just that in order to scare pregnant women into following doctors' orders.

When I was pregnant in 2002 with my oldest son, I dutifully bought a copy of the best-selling *What to Expect When You're Expecting* and attempted to follow a diet high in calcium, lean protein, leafy green vegetables, whole grains, and vitamin C, and low in salt, sugar, caffeine, and alcohol. The authors, Arlene Eisenberg, Heidi Murkoff, and Sandee Hathaway, promised that if I followed all their dietary rules in their "Best-Odds," I would "come as close as possible to guaranteeing [my] baby not just good health, but excellent health."[56] They claimed the authority of science, citing a study of the relationship between diet during pregnancy and newborn health conducted at the Harvard School of Public Health. "Of the women in the study whose diets were good to excellent, fully 95% had babies in good or excellent health. On the other hand, only 8% of women whose diets were really awful (composed largely of junk foods) had babies in good or excellent health, and 65% of them had infants who were stillborn, premature, functionally immature, or who had congenital defects."[57] This statement is every bit as alarmist, and every bit as thin on evidence, as Evans's claim that a woman can cause Down syndrome in her baby by eating "red meats, eggs, fish, chicken and highly seasoned foods."

Like authors before them, Eisenberg, Murkoff, and Hathaway advocated sacrifice and self-discipline:

> You've got only nine months of meals and snacks with which to give your baby the best possible start in life. Make every one of them count. Before you close your mouth on a forkful of food, consider, "Is this the best bite I can give my baby?" If it will benefit your baby, chew away. If it'll only benefit your sweet tooth or appease your appetite, put your fork down.[58]

All of this advice reflects changing medical ideas as well as cultural and geographic differences in diet and activities. Avicenna specifically recommends two Persian dishes—"alesfidabegi," which is a "lamb stew with coriander," and "al-zerbeiet" (or "zerbagi"), a porridge with cumin, sugar, almonds, and vinegar—as ideal for pregnant women.[59] West's insistence on fresh air was typical of public health advice in the early twentieth-century US. Keeping bedroom windows open at night in all seasons and houses well-aired were hygienic practices urged on all Americans.[60] Eisenberg, Murkoff, and Hathaway opined that if a pregnant woman planned to eat out, her healthiest restaurant options were "American, continental, and steak houses."[61]

While some of this older advice for pregnant women might amuse modern readers, we do well to bear in mind that much of the advice about nutrition and exercise given to pregnant women today is based on sketchy science and unacknowledged cultural preferences. As Emily Oster points out, the advice commonly given to pregnant women in America to avoid alcohol, caffeine, sushi, hair dye, and changing cat litter has little to no evidentiary basis.[62] Further, advice to pregnant women varies considerably across the world.[63] American women are strictly enjoined never to eat raw fish while pregnant. Japanese women are told that raw fish is "part of good neonatal nutrition."[64] American women are told that saunas and hot tubs are dangerous to pregnant women and their babies. Finnish women use saunas throughout their pregnancies and even give birth in them. American women are advised to give up bicycling while pregnant because of the risk of falling. Danish women, many of whom do not own cars, continue to cycle all through their pregnancies and have even been known to cycle to the hospital when they go into labor. Recommendations about alcohol, caffeine, unpasteurized cheese, and even fresh fruit and vegetables vary from country to country across the world, even within "Western" countries that share traditions of biomedicine.[65]

Two things have remained constant through changing medical fashions and cultural iterations. The first is the premise that pregnant women need to follow a diet and exercise regimen prescribed by (mostly male) medical authorities. And a corollary of this premise is that failure to follow this advice can have devastating and lifelong consequences for the fetus. Whether the child is born with an "ignoble soul," as Soranus warned, or saddled with "worse odds" in the game of life, the message is clear that bad decisions during pregnancy can cause irreversible harm to the fetus.

The second constant in pregnancy advice since antiquity is that the majority of the recommendations for diet and exercise can be followed only by women with significant resources of time, money, and social status. Soranus suggested that pregnant women have their slaves carry them around in sedan chairs, get regular massages, and eat expensive delicacies. As Anna Bonnell Freidin points out, Soranus's assertion that a baby whose mother did not or could not follow all of his recommendations for diet and lifestyle would have a "misshapen" body and an "ignoble soul" implied that only the children of the elite would have beautiful bodies and noble souls.[66] In general, Avicenna advised pregnant women to avoid drugs, which could harm the fetus. If they needed something to settle their stomachs, however, he recommended an "electuary" made of a perfect, unblemished pearl ground up with spices including pepper, cardamom, nutmeg, cinnamon, and sugar. It goes without saying that crushed pearls and imported spices were not available to all women in tenth-century Persia. Avicenna and Savonarola advised pregnant women to eat bread made from wheat rather than bread made from coarser grains like bran. Savonarola noted that poor women could not eat bread made with the more expensive wheat flour and had to subsist on bread made from cheaper, coarser grains. But he concluded that because poor women were accustomed to this diet, it was less harmful to their babies than it would be to wealthy women. And while he recommended that elite women take very light exercise while pregnant, he believed that peasant women "benefit from the great exercise they do."[67] In other words, the bodies of the poor were coarser and hardier than the refined and elegant bodies of the rich, and these class differences were passed from mother to child. Ironically, in the twentieth and twenty-first centuries, when whole-grain and "artisanal" breads became more expensive than white bread, these recommendations flipped. The authors of *What to Expect* urged women to steer clear of white than the price of junk food.[70] The high cost of healthy food is one of the major reasons that obesity and poverty are so strongly correlated.[71]

I spent both of my pregnancies in Oklahoma, where fifty-four of the seventy-seven counties, including the one in which I live, contain food deserts. A food desert is an area in which a significant percentage of the population does not have ready access to grocery stores where they can purchase fresh fruits and vegetables.[72] For many pregnant women in my state, fresh fruit and vegetables are as inaccessible as Persian electuaries made of crushed pearls. And yet public law and policy in Oklahoma, as in many other states, continues to hold mothers responsible for poor birth outcomes. Oklahoma is a state with poor infant and maternal mortality rates. Its efforts to improve the health of fetuses and neonates focus on educating mothers about diet and exercise, smoking, and the benefits of breastfeeding. There have been few attempts to make structural changes to ensure that all mothers have access to healthy food, clean water, and a safe and unpolluted environment in which to gestate their babies and raise their children.

The case of Brittney Poolaw, with which I began this chapter, exemplifies the difference between the real and the imagined risks to fetuses. Poolaw is Native American. She lives in Comanche County, Oklahoma, a predominantly rural area in the southwest of the state. These two facts about Poolaw—that she is Native American and that she lives in rural Oklahoma—both put her at higher risk for poor outcomes the minute she got pregnant. Both are considerably bigger risk factors for preterm birth, low birth weight, neonatal death, and maternal death than marijuana and methamphetamine use. Native American women have higher rates of preterm birth (defined as birth before thirty-seven-weeks gestation), higher rates of miscarriages, and higher rates of maternal death than the national average.[73] Native American infants have higher rates of death than the national average. These dismal statistics are part of a long and ugly history of attacks on the reproductive autonomy of Native women, a history that includes coercive sterilization and the forced removal of Native children to boarding schools and foster care.

Poolaw's location also put her at increased risk for pregnancy complications. About 17 percent of the population of Comanche County is below the poverty line,[74] and about 13 percent have no health insurance.[75] Almost 60 percent of the population of Comanche County lives a significant distance from a grocery store, making fresh, healthy food difficult to access.[76] The infant mortality rate in Comanche County is 8.90 deaths per 1,000 births, higher than the state rate of 7.70 per 1,000, which is in turn higher than the national rate of 5.79 per 1,000. Oklahoma has the fourth-worst maternal mortality rate in the country, behind Alabama, Kentucky, and Arkansas.[77] Access to health care in general and to reproductive services in particular is poor.[78]

The ability to eat a healthy diet, get the right amount and kind of physical activity, and to avoid situations and substances that are harmful to the fetus has always been dependent on socioeconomic status. And yet, when women fail to follow the accepted pregnancy regimen, they are blamed for their individual failure. In the United States we have yet to see sweeping policy changes that would allow all pregnant people to follow a healthy diet and exercise regimen. Such policies would include not only those traditionally linked to the health of women and children such as mandatory paid maternity leave and universal health care covering prenatal care and childbirth but also policies that would make healthy foods readily accessible to all. And as long as we remain convinced that the major threats to fetuses come from the women who carry them, we never will.

PUNISHING PREGNANT WOMEN

All of the advice on what to eat and what to do while pregnant strongly suggests that poor pregnancy outcomes—including miscarriages, stillbirths, and disabled infants—are the fault of the mother. Almost everything that can go wrong with a pregnancy goes wrong because the mother fails to eat the right foods, drink the right beverages, get the right exercise, and maintain a calm and happy state of mind. Or worse, things go wrong because the mother has consumed the wrong substances, indulged in dangerous activities, or become angry or depressed. The burden of a successful birth—a full-term, healthy, beautiful, intelligent baby—is almost entirely on the mother. Or at least, that is what we are led to believe.

Perhaps the starkest evidence for the persistence of the old idea that the womb is a dangerous place is to be found in the hysteria surrounding pregnant women like Poolaw who use drugs, especially but not exclusively illegal drugs. In the 1980s and 1990s there was public furor over Black women who smoked crack cocaine while pregnant. These women were demonized and accused of producing "crack babies," children who were permanently disabled and would grow up to be burdens to society. As the *New York Times* editorial board admitted in 2018, "*The New York Times, The Washington Post, Time, Newsweek* and others further demonized black women 'addicts' by wrongly reporting that they were giving birth to a generation of neurologically damaged children who were less than fully human and who would bankrupt the schools and social service agencies once they came of age."[79]

Newborns who tested positive for cocaine were taken away from their mothers and placed in foster care. Even at the time, the evidence that cocaine caused severe neurological problems, delayed physical development, long-term cognitive deficits, and behavioral problems was thin at best. Since the 2000s it has become abundantly clear that the dangers of prenatal exposure to cocaine were vastly overestimated. As Jeanne Flavin writes, "In contrast to the devastating impact [of prenatal cocaine exposure] predicted by sensationalist media accounts, meta-analyses (i.e., studies of many other studies) found small or no effects on physical growth, cognition, language skills, motor skills, behavior, attention, affect, and neurophysiology."[80] Given appropriate treatment, the overwhelming majority of babies born with cocaine in their systems recover and develop normally with no long-term effects. Health problems in babies of women addicted to crack were the result of poverty and racism and were exacerbated by policies of separating mothers and babies.

Although the myth of the "crack baby" has been debunked, new fears of the dangers of methamphetamine and opioids to fetuses have fueled more prosecutions of women. There have been hundreds of cases in which pregnant women have been arrested and imprisoned for drug use and had their babies taken away. In a great many of these cases, infants were born healthy, and there was no evidence that prenatal drug exposure caused any lasting harm.[81] A ProPublica study conducted in 2015 found that "at least 479 new and expecting mothers have been prosecuted across Alabama since 2006." Examples include a woman who took a small amount of Valium while pregnant, no trace of which showed up in her perfectly healthy newborn's system; a woman with epilepsy who substituted marijuana for her anti-seizure medications because marijuana posed less of a risk to her fetus; and a woman who took methadone prescribed by a doctor.[82] Again, the moral indignation heaped on women who use illicit drugs while pregnant is out of all proportion to the actual risks to the fetus.[83]

The prosecution of women who use drugs while pregnant is certainly a product of the growing belief that the fetus is a person whose rights must be protected. But the willingness of doctors, nurses, police, prosecutors, social workers, juries, and journalists to believe that illicit drugs cause inevitable and irreparable damage to fetuses is also rooted in the much older idea that the womb is a dangerous place.

MATERNAL EMOTIONS

In the early twentieth century, the notion of maternal imagination came under increasing criticism from obstetricians and embryologists, but the notion that maternal emotions, especially anger, stress, and depression, could harm the fetus has remained constant. Franklin Mall, professor of anatomy at the Johns Hopkins School of Medicine and one of the country's leading embryologists, ridiculed "the theory of maternal impresses" as "futile speculations over mere coincidences."[84] This view was echoed in popular pregnancy guides and in syndicated newspaper health columns. West informed her readers that "doctors and other scientists are now practically agreed that [maternal impressions] have no basis in fact."[85] Charles Reed, a Chicago obstetrician who authored *What Every Expectant Mother Should Know* (1924), stated baldly: "The scientific fact is that it is impossible for the mother to mark her off-spring, either intentionally or by accident."[86] In a column in the *Los Angeles Times* in 1932, the physician William Brady answered the question "Are Babies 'Marked' By Prenatal Influence?" with a resounding negative. He characterized this belief as "one of the cruelest superstitions prevailing among the ignorant and the misinformed" and one that caused expectant mothers "much needless anxiety and worry."[87] He took up the topic of maternal impression again in 1947 in his syndicated "Here's to Health" column, arguing that "embryology should be taught in high school" in order to dispel the myth of maternal imagination. "No one who has an elementary knowledge of embryology can entertain for an instant any such old wives' tale," he asserted. These repeated assertions from doctors and public health officials demonstrate that maternal imagination had fallen out of favor with the scientifically inclined or trained, but also that the idea hung on a long time. Well into the twentieth century, authors advising pregnant women felt they had to counter this notion. However, their ongoing concern that mothers control their emotions during pregnancy, that they remain calm and cheerful, belies the seemingly clear repudiation of maternal impressions. As maternal imagination faded from science it was replaced by concerns about "stress" and "worry" during pregnancy and their impact on the fetus.

In his *Mother, Nurse, and Infant* of 1889, the physician S. P. Sackett wrote:

A tranquil mind is of the greatest importance. Forebodings of a gloomy nature should not be encouraged, as they often are, by relating dismal stories, etc. Unnecessary fear upon the part of the mother may have a bad effect upon the child, as may also the indulgence in unbridled anger, or yielding to temper,—perhaps may cause convulsions or hemorrhage, or even abortion. There is reason to believe that the imagination of the mother has an influence on the beauty of the child; and it is quite certain that cheerfulness and equanimity of mind contributes to the future good health of the child, and may even affect its disposition and mental traits.[88]

Within two decades, most doctors would stoutly deny that "the imagination of the mother has an influence on the beauty of the child." However, doctors and other pregnancy experts continued to believe that a mother's emotions were communicated to the fetus in utero. Gloominess, fear, and anger could harm the fetus and even cause a miscarriage. Tranquility, cheerfulness, and equanimity created a healthy environment for the fetus to grow and develop.

By the early twentieth century, advice to pregnant women simultaneously denied the influence of maternal imagination and reaffirmed the importance of maintaining a proper emotional state. The notion that the mother's emotional state during pregnancy could affect her baby lingered on long after maternal imagination died. West, for example, chided the pregnant woman who "goes through her pregnancy repining or lamenting her condition."[89] And the obstetrician Charles Reed opined that "the mental condition should be placid without either excitement or depression."[90]

While "maternal imagination" is no longer a medical category, the idea that mothers' emotional states pose a threat to their fetuses has continued to permeate our culture. Medical and nursing journals contain a plethora of articles with titles like "Prenatal Stress and Depression Associated Neuronal Development in Neonates," "Effects of Maternal Prenatal Stress on Offspring Development," "Stress during Pregnancy and Epigenetic Modifications to Offspring DNA," and "Relation of Outbursts of Anger and the Acute Risk of Placental Abruption."[91] I am not denying that emotions can have real physiological effects on the body and that in pregnant women these might impact the fetus. But emotions do not occur in a social or cultural vacuum. Serenity, patience, and cheerfulness have long been considered desirable qualities in women, especially mothers, especially when coupled with obedience to medical authority. By contrast, anger has long been considered an inappropriate and unattractive emotion for women, especially Black women.[92] Further, just as the ability to eat a healthy diet and perform the right kind of physical activity is closely tied to socioeconomic status, so too is the ability to manage stress.[93] The higher up in the social hierarchy a woman is embedded, the less likely she is to experience stress, anxiety, depression, and irritability. The lower down the social ladder she finds herself, the more likely she is to experience these negative emotions.

To illustrate the continuities in thinking about the dangers of maternal emotions, let me juxtapose two cases of maternal anger from two different centuries. The first comes from the casebooks of the eighteenth-century German physician Johann Storch, as analyzed by the historian Barbara Duden. In November 1735, Storch examined an "unmarried pregnant person" who had been badly beaten by a young man and was in danger of miscarrying. Storch attributed the threat of miscarriage to the woman's great anger and vexation over the fight, not to the effect of the beating itself.[94]

The second case is much more recent. On December 4, 2018, a twenty-seven-year-old Alabama woman named Marshae Jones, who was five months pregnant, got into a physical altercation with her coworker, twenty-three-year-old Ebony Jemison. In the course of this fight, Jemison took out a gun and shot Jones in the belly. Jones survived the shooting, but her unborn baby did not. Although Jemison was arrested immediately after the shooting, it was Jones who was ultimately indicted for manslaughter in the death of her fetus. A grand jury decided that Jones was responsible because she "initiat[ed] a fight knowing she was five months pregnant." In the face of national criticism over a woman being prosecuted for a pregnancy loss after she was shot, District Attorney Lynneice Washington dismissed the charges.[95] This case made painfully clear the ways in which treating the fetus as a person can have dire consequences for pregnant women, even those like Marshae Jones, who had no intention of terminating her pregnancy. But the willingness of the police and grand jury members to believe that Marshae Jones caused her fetus's death because she could not control her anger stands in a long tradition of blaming fetal death and miscarriage on women's emotions. Like the unnamed "unmarried pregnant person" in Johann Storch's account two hundred years earlier, the injuries Jones sustained at the hands of another are less relevant to why she lost her pregnancy than her own emotional state.

ENVIRONMENTAL HARMS

There is overwhelming evidence that exposure to chemicals and heavy metals in utero poses far greater risks to the life and health of fetuses than maternal diet and behavior during pregnancy. Flint, Michigan, provides a recent and tragic example of the dangers of prenatal exposure to lead. Up until April 2014, the city of Flint received water pumped from Lake Huron by the Detroit Water and Sewerage Department. In April, as a cost-saving measure, the city's emergency manager switched the water source to the Flint River. Although Flint residents noticed that the water was no longer clear and had an unpleasant odor, their complaints were dismissed by the city administration. Residents were repeatedly assured that the water was safe, despite mounting evidence that it contained multiple dangerous contaminants. Finally in August 2015, a research team from Virginia Polytechnic Institute and State University reported high levels of lead in the Flint water supply. In September, Flint pediatrician Mona Hanna-Attisha reported finding substantially elevated blood lead levels in children. The city initially sought to deny these reports, but it finally switched back to Lake Huron water on October 16, 2015.

The health consequences of the high lead levels in the Flint water supply have been catastrophic and are still being untangled. But here I focus on one particular set of consequences: the lead in the Flint water had devastating consequences for fetal life and health. At least two separate studies have shown that the number of babies in Flint born with low birth weight increased during the period in which the water supply was contaminated with lead.[96] Even more strikingly, the number of babies born to women in Flint dropped appreciably compared to women in other parts of Michigan. The most plausible explanation of this drop in the birth rate is "fetal death and miscarriage." The authors sum up their results: "The population of women aged 15–49 in Flint during our study period is approximately 26,000. The GFR [general fertility rate] dropped from 62 to 57 [births per 1,000 women], suggesting that over our study window of 17 months (births conceived from November 2013 through March 2015), between 198 and 276 more children would have been born had Flint not switched its water source."[97]

The increase in fetal deaths in Flint is tragic but completely consistent with numerous other studies. For example, Marc Edwards also documented a "higher incidence of miscarriages and fetal death" in his study of Washington, DC, during the drinking water "lead crisis" from 2000 to 2004.[98] Grossman and Slusky note that, despite the clear evidence of harm to fetuses from exposure to lead, the Trump administration called "for a substantial decrease in funding for the EPA, which is charged with ensuring that localities maintain minimum water standards."[99]

In addition to lead, there is ample empirical evidence that a range of other environmental toxins cause irreparable damage to fetuses in utero, as well as to children and adults. Native American reservations in the western United States have suffered severe heavy metal contamination from abandoned uranium mines for years. Infant mortality rates among Native Americans are 28 percent higher than in non-Hispanic whites, and rates of birth defects are 50 percent higher. These rates are not all attributable to heavy metal contamination; a lack of safe drinking water and soil contamination are also linked to a wide range of health problems on reservations.[100]

The Center for the Health Assessment of Mothers and Children of Salinas (CHAMACOS) Study, begun in 1999, is a study of the impact of pesticides and other chemicals among the children of agricultural workers.[101] This study has found an association between prenatal exposure to organophosphate pesticides and "adverse neurological effects, including loss of IQ, cognitive deficits, behavioral issues like lack of attention, and respiratory problems." Over twenty separate studies have found a link between fetal exposure to organophosphate pesticides and long-term, permanent neurological damage. Despite these findings, the Environmental Protection Agency has refused to issue bans or even warnings about the use of these chemicals.[102]

Hydraulic fracturing—commonly known as "fracking"—is a process used to extract gas and oil from shale rock. Fracking provides cheap electricity and avoids the air pollution and carbon emissions that accompany other forms of fuel extraction. However, fracking is far more dangerous than the oil and gas industry admit, especially to children born near fracking sites. In fracking, liquid is injected into rock at high pressure, and this forces out the oil and gas. The chemicals used in fracking operations are toxic, and they regularly contaminate water supplies, including the drinking water, of nearby communities. Multiple studies have demonstrated the health hazards of living near fracking sites, including harm to fetuses. Rates of miscarriage are significantly higher near fracking sites. And newborns in these areas are more likely to be underweight and to suffer from other health problems.[103]

And yet, instead of focusing on environmental hazards like these that pose such risks to fetuses, or ensuring that all pregnant women have access to healthy food, clean water, safe neighborhoods, and high-quality medical care, our elected representatives, obstetricians, prosecutors, and police consistently seek to protect them from their mothers. Miscarriages are treated as suspicious deaths rather than personal tragedies. Substance abuse and addiction are treated like child abuse rather than medical problems. Pregnant women are subjected to intrusive investigations and invasive medical procedures. None of this has had a positive impact on the health and well-being of fetuses; if anything, it has harmed fetuses. These actions perpetuate a culture that has treated pregnant mothers suspiciously for thousands of years. There are real and present dangers to fetuses, but these dangers do not come from their mothers.

4

THE SECRETS OF WOMEN

In 2015, Mark Zuckerberg announced on Facebook that he and his wife Priscilla Chan were expecting their first child. He also revealed that they had suffered three miscarriages prior to this pregnancy, stating that he and Chan hoped that sharing their experience would "help more people feel comfortable sharing their stories as well." Zuckerberg and Chan were widely praised for speaking openly about their difficulties starting a family. Numerous articles following the couple's statement discussed the prevalence of miscarriage, pointing out that almost all women who have been pregnant or who have tried to get pregnant have had at least one miscarriage, whether they realize it or not.[1] In the years since Zuckerberg's post, other celebrities have shared their stories of pregnancy loss, catalyzing an increase in public discussions of what not long ago was considered a private and almost taboo topic.

In September 2018, country music singer Carrie Underwood told *People* magazine that she had had three miscarriages over the previous two years.[2] Since then Underwood has spoken about her miscarriages several times in interviews and in a short film she made with her husband Mike Fisher.[3] She describes feeling guilt and shame, agonizing over why her body was not "doing something it was 'supposed to do,'" and wondering if she had done something wrong.[4] But she also asserted that miscarriages should not be "a dirty secret."[5] Again, many of the interviews and articles about Underwood's miscarriages included information about the prevalence of miscarriages and praised Underwood for sharing her experiences.

In November 2020, Meghan Markle wrote an editorial in the *New York Times* revealing that she had suffered a miscarriage in July.[6] Like Zuckerberg and Underwood, she described the isolation that comes from experiencing a kind of loss that is not supposed to be discussed publicly:

> Losing a child means carrying an almost unbearable grief, experienced by many but talked about by few. In the pain of our loss, my husband and I discovered that in a room of 100 women, 10 to 20 of them will have suffered from miscarriage. Yet despite the staggering commonality of this pain, the conversation remains taboo, riddled with (unwarranted) shame, and perpetuating a cycle of solitary mourning.

Markle, too, was praised for her openness about her pregnancy loss.

There is a constant refrain in these stories: no one talks about miscarriage—until you have one, and only then do you learn how common they are. A miscarriage is an initiation into a club that you never knew existed and never wanted to join. But only when you are a member will people talk openly about miscarriage with you. The secrecy and taboo surrounding pregnancy loss contribute to feelings of shame and guilt. When you do not realize how common miscarriages are, it can feel like you must have done something wrong, a feeling exacerbated by the medical and social tendency to blame women for poor pregnancy outcomes.

All three of these miscarriage stories are strikingly different from Brittney Poolaw's story, with which I began the last chapter, or from any of the stories of women prosecuted for miscarriages that I discussed. Celebrity miscarriage stories are always about women who wanted to be pregnant, women who did the "right" things: consulted doctors and followed their advice, took prenatal vitamins, ate organic foods, eliminated (or at least cut back on) alcohol and caffeine, took yoga classes, and practiced mindfulness. These are women with financial security, access to excellent health care, and supportive partners. The responses to celebrity miscarriages are almost uniformly sympathetic. Many people seem willing to grant sympathy to women they perceive as "good mothers," women they believe did everything they could to stay pregnant and who mourn their "lost children." But for women who will not or cannot present themselves as "good mothers," the responses are frighteningly unsympathetic. Women who express any ambivalence about being pregnant, who lack access to health care and healthy food, or who struggle with drug or alcohol addiction are treated very differently when their pregnancies end in miscarriage. And those who simply do not look like good mothers because they are young, single, poor, Black, Hispanic, or Indigenous also do not get sympathy when their pregnancies end in miscarriage.

These two kinds of miscarriage stories are linked. Both reflect a tendency to blame women for pregnancy loss. The first set of stories illustrates the tendency of women to blame themselves, to question whether they—inadvertently—did something to terminate their own pregnancies. The second set illustrates a willingness—on the part of medical practitioners, prosecutors, judges, juries, and the general public—to believe that some women intentionally cause their own miscarriages. Both these attitudes are irrational. Approximately one in five pregnancies ends in miscarriage, and most miscarriages are caused by genetic abnormalities in the fetus.

Media coverage of celebrity miscarriages always emphasizes that miscarriages are common, that most cases have nothing to do with any actions the pregnant person took or did not take, and that most women who miscarry will go on to have successful pregnancies. And yet the constant expressions of guilt, the constant need to repeat that miscarriage is not a "dirty secret" and that the shame is unwarranted, insidiously suggest that these really are the only appropriate emotions when dealing with a miscarriage. Grief and guilt are "natural" and "normal" when dealing with the loss of a "child."

Shannon Withycombe points out that women who express relief or indifference when they miscarry frequently face disapproval, as if those emotions are callous or wrong. When blogger Penelope Trunk announced on Twitter that she was having a miscarriage, she added: "Thank goodness, because there's a fucked-up 3-week hoop-jump to have an abortion in Wisconsin."[7] Trunk, unlike Zuckerberg, Underwood, and Markle, was not praised for her frank and public discussion of miscarriage or for challenging an outdated taboo. Instead, she was accused of insensitivity for her cavalier attitude toward the loss of a "human being" and for expressing relief "about something that devastates other women."[8] "While we may be in a new age of miscarriage openness," Withycombe comments, "so far the most appropriate miscarriage discussion is one that revolves around loss, sadness, and grief."[9] Given that about half of all pregnancies are unplanned, it stands to reason that at least some pregnant people would respond to a miscarriage with relief and would not perceive it as the loss of a baby. And yet this kind of miscarriage story is rarely aired in public.

One of the pieces of evidence used against Poolaw in her manslaughter trial was that she told a police detective who questioned her after her miscarriage that "when she found out she was pregnant she didn't know if she wanted the baby or not."[10] It should go without saying that not wanting to be pregnant does not cause or even increase the likelihood of a miscarriage. But in states like Oklahoma that have enacted near total bans on abortion after the overturning of *Roe v. Wade,* and where any pregnancy loss can be investigated as a possible abortion, women expressing relief at the ending of an unwanted pregnancy—to a friend or a medical practitioner, or on social media—could very easily face prosecution.

Why, despite all we know about the frequency of early pregnancy loss and its causes, are we collectively unable to treat miscarriage as a normal part of reproductive life? Why do we persist in believing that women are to blame for miscarriages?

Part of the answer to these questions lies in the very recent past and the efforts of the pro-life movement to ascribe personhood to every fertilized egg, so that any pregnancy termination, spontaneous or induced, is the death of a "baby." The historians Lara Freidenfelds and Shannon Withycombe found that in the eighteenth- and nineteenth-century United States, women and their partners did not always respond with grief to early miscarriages. Many women took them in stride as a normal part of their reproductive lives. If they had several successful pregnancies, resulting in live births, they were unlikely to be especially bothered by a few lost pregnancies. Some even responded with relief if they thought the pregnancy might threaten their health, especially if it came very soon after the birth of another child.[11] This changed as middle-class families began trying to limit family size, investing more emotional and financial resources in fewer children.

Only in the late twentieth century have women been encouraged to "bond" with their "baby" the moment they see a positive result on a pregnancy test, something that makes early miscarriages much more emotionally fraught than they used to be.[12]

But another part of the answer lies in the much more distant past. I traced the long history of seeing the womb as a dangerous place, of women endangering their fetuses because they are irrational and emotional. Here I follow a darker strand in the history of reproduction: the belief that women are inherently evil and deliberately harm the fetuses in their wombs. Since the ancient Greeks, medical writers have asserted that women can tell they are pregnant from the moment they conceive. They have also claimed that the fetus is only loosely attached to the womb in the first two or three months of pregnancy and easily shaken loose. Some women take advantage of this fact and deliberately cause miscarriage by moving vigorously—jumping, dancing, or having sex. Women who can tell they are pregnant well before there are any visible signs of pregnancy can rid themselves of unwanted pregnancies without their husbands, lovers, or physicians being any the wiser.

The figure of the malicious woman, sexually voracious and skilled in the arts of contraception and abortion, who kills her innocent fetus, or helps other women kill their fetuses, can be traced from the ancient Greeks into the twenty-first century. She emerges particularly vividly in a medieval book called *On the Secrets of Women*. This book was written by a German monk around 1300. In the preface, he claimed that he wrote for a fellow monk who had asked him "to bring to light certain hidden, secret things about that nature of women."[13] Although the identity of this monk is unknown, *On the Secrets of Women* continued to be read and studied for the next three hundred years.

The phrase "secrets of women" was used by many medieval authors.[14] According to historians Katharine Park and Monica Green, the phrase has at least two connotations. First, "women's secrets" meant information about human reproduction, about the processes of conception, fetal development, and birth that went on in the female body. In this sense, women and women's bodies were the objects of knowledge. Second, "women's secrets" could be things women knew about sex and procreation that they kept secret from men. In this sense, women were possessors of "a body of secret knowledge about sexuality and generation."[15] The second meaning of "women's secrets" implied that women were naturally malicious and evil, using knowledge of sex and procreation to do harm and further their own ends. It was important for men to learn "women's secrets" so they could see through female deception and foil feminine schemes. Both meanings are intertwined in *On the Secrets of Women*. The author describes how the male and female seeds unite in the uterus. He details how the planets and the sun and moon influence the development of the fetus. He explains how lactating women produce milk. But he also claims that women know ways to trick men or to hurt them. Women pretend to be virgins when they are not, for example, or they place iron in their vaginas and have sex with men while the moon is waning which causes "a large wound and a serious infection of the penis."[16]

It will come as no great surprise that a medieval monk living and writing in a celibate, all-male milieu would be virulently misogynistic and that his book on reproduction would be filled with fear and loathing of women. I begin with him, not because he is typical—his positions are in many cases extreme—but because he makes explicit what many other authors leave implicit. The author of *On the Secrets of Women* believed that women could tell they were pregnant as soon as they conceived and that they could use this knowledge to abort their fetuses before any man was even aware that they were pregnant.

Let us focus first on the idea that women can tell if they are pregnant or not as soon as they have sex. Our German monk lists multiple "signs of conception." Some of them are familiar to us today: missed menstrual period and desire for "unusual foods." These signs could be seen and understood by the woman, but also by those around her. But the two earliest signs occur immediately following the sexual act and can be sensed only by the woman. The first sign is that the "woman feels cold and has pain in her legs immediately after coitus with a man." The second is that very little of the man's semen falls out of the woman's vagina after intercourse.[17] The text offers one sign of conception that could be sensed by the man alone: "If the man feels his penis drawn and sucked into the closure of the vulva" during sex, this indicated that the woman had conceived.[18] These signs of pregnancy were based on a particular understanding of the mechanics of conception. They were based on the notion that both men and women have "seed" and that during intercourse both ejaculate seed into the woman's uterus. Conception occurred when the two seeds combined: "And after these seeds are received, the womb closes up like a purse on every side, so that nothing can fall out of it."[19] It was this closing of the womb that women, and sometimes men, could allegedly feel immediately after (productive) sex. Because the womb was then shut tight, none of the man's semen fell out of the vagina after sex. The sensation of cold was caused by the womb drawing heat to itself, heat that was necessary to nurture the combined seed as it developed. Concentrating heat in the womb left other parts of the body cold.

Because women, according to our monk, generally knew they were pregnant before their male partner or medical practitioner did, and because the embryo was most vulnerable to miscarriage early in pregnancy, it was eminently possible for women to rid themselves of unwanted pregnancies. The embryo was only loosely attached to the womb in the first weeks of pregnancy and could easily be shaken loose by vigorous movement or lifting heavy weights or even a jarring carriage ride. As we have seen, pregnant women were advised to avoid these activities and a host of others that were thought to be dangerous to the fetus. But this knowledge could be turned to nefarious purposes. According to our monk, "prostitutes and women learned in the [art of abortion] engage in a good deal of activity when they are pregnant," including traveling, dancing, wrestling, and having sex, in order to rid themselves of unwanted pregnancies.[20]

It would clearly be advantageous to men to be able to discern if a woman is pregnant, so they can prevent her from harming the fetus. Our monk provides such a test. If you want to find out whether a woman is pregnant, he writes, "give her hydromel [a mixture of water and honey] to drink." This concoction causes cramps in the belly if she is pregnant. However, the monk warns that some women are sneaky and dishonest. If you tell them you are giving them a pregnancy test, they will lie to you about the cramps. He suggests that men employ trickery: "Wait until the woman complains of pain in the head or somewhere else, as women are accustomed to do, and then give her the drink as a remedy against it." Then ask her "if she has pain anywhere," and see what she says. If "she says she feels discomfort around the umbilicus," then you know she is pregnant. If she says she has no pain, or pain somewhere else in her body, then you know she is not pregnant. But he cautions, "Some women, however, are so clever and so aware of the trick that they refuse to tell the truth, but rather say something else instead."[21] In the end, men must rely on women to give an accurate description of their bodily sensations in order to determine whether they are pregnant.

The notion that when conception occurs the womb closes tight to hold in the seed, and that women could feel this happening and thus know the instant they were pregnant, can be traced back to the ancient Greeks. It was repeated in medical literature for the next two millennia and retains a hold to this day. In the Hippocratic treatise *On the Nature of the Child*, one of the earliest and most influential writings on pregnancy and fetal development, we read that "when a woman is about to conceive, the seed does not run out of her, but remains inside." The author claims this is something women can feel immediately and a fact women tell each other about pregnancy.[22] The framing of this "fact" as something "women say" about reproduction and that women share with each other should be taken with several large grains of salt. But it was a very influential claim. For the next two thousand years, medical authors agreed that women knew they were pregnant as soon as they conceived.

The Roman physician Soranus also gave a list of signs of conception in his *Gynecology*. These included "a shivering sensation" felt by the woman after intercourse. He also noted that if a woman had conceived, the seed would be retained in the uterus, and thus "the vagina is not kept moist by the seed or only slightly."[23] According to the sixteenth-century physician Jacques Guillemeau, if after sex her partner's semen did not fall out of her and if she felt "a shaking or quivering" and a chill, this indicated pregnancy. Like the author of *On the Secrets of Women*, he asserted that if a man felt "a kind of sucking or drawing at the end of his yard [penis]" after ejaculation, then he might confidently inform his partner that she was pregnant.[24] The seventeenth-century midwife Jane Sharp also says the first sign that a woman is pregnant is, "if when the seed is cast into the womb, she feel the womb shut close, and a shivering or trembling to run through every part of her body, and that is by reason of the heat that draws inward to keep the conception, and so leaves the outward parts cold & chill." Further, when a woman has conceived, "the mans seed comes not forth again, for the womb closely embraceth it, and will shut as fast as possibly may be."[25] On into the eighteenth century, the wildly popular guide to sex and procreation *Aristotle's Masterpiece*, stated that "a Coldness and Chilness of the outward Parts after Copulation, shews a Woman to have conceived; the Heat being retired to make the Conception."[26]

All this talk of shivering, quivering, shaking, and trembling might suggest that these authors were talking about female orgasms. But most are clear that the shivering comes *after* the sexual act and is caused, not by pleasure, but by the sudden cold caused by the withdrawal of body heat into the womb. However, most medical authors held that female pleasure was essential for conception. Pleasure was what caused the female body to emit seed, in the same way that pleasure caused the male body to ejaculate. As the author of *On the Secrets of Women* put it: "When a woman is having sex with a man she experiences such a great pleasure from the male member rubbing back and forth on the nerves and veins in the vagina that the vagina dilates and ejects the menses [seed]." Only if a woman experienced pleasure during intercourse would her body emit the seed necessary to form a fetus. Both female and male orgasm were synonymous with the emission of seed. Ideally, the emission of seed from the male and female partners—their orgasms—should be simultaneous. Every pregnancy required a male orgasm, and by the logic of this view of conception, every pregnancy also required a female orgasm. For a woman to be pregnant, she had to have emitted seed during intercourse. This meant that pregnancy itself was evidence of female orgasm.

Numerous medical authors claimed that women enjoyed sex more than men because they derived pleasure both from emitting their own seed and from receiving the male seed, whereas men only experienced the pleasure of emitting their own seed.[27] Some authors, like Guillemeau, claimed that it was a sign of pregnancy if a woman derived exceptional pleasure from sex, which reflects the view that simultaneous orgasms were necessary for conception and that women derive pleasure both from their own emission of seed and from the reception of their partner's.

The belief that simultaneous orgasms were necessary for conception might seem to be one that would be easily disproved by experience. Shouldn't it have been obvious to people in the past, as it is to us today, that women could get pregnant without enjoying sex, let alone having an orgasm? But the myth of the necessity of simultaneous orgasms for conception hung on in obstetrical texts into the nineteenth and twentieth centuries. Prominent professors of obstetrics affirmed that simultaneous orgasms were necessary for conception or, at least, rendered conception more probable.

Barton Cooke Hirst (1861–1935), professor of obstetrics at the University of Pennsylvania, stated: "The orgasm of male and female should be synchronous; as the seminal fluid is ejaculated from the penis it is sucked in part into the uterine cavity."[28] And James Clifton Edgar (1859–1939), professor of obstetrics at Cornell University Medical College, taught that "the orgasm is the climax of the sexual act. Its normal occurrence is simultaneous in the male and female, and makes conception more probable."[29] The idea retains some currency today. In *What to Expect When You're Expecting* Heidi Murkoff notes that "some women 'feel' they're pregnant within days—even moments—of conception."[30] The longevity of this myth reflects the deep distrust of women that is so clearly expressed in the *Secrets of Women*. Women's accounts of their own bodily experiences are not to be trusted. Women lie, especially when it comes to matters of sex and reproduction.

The belief in the necessity of female pleasure for conception underlay the view that pregnancy could not result from rape. Pregnancy was evidence of orgasm, and orgasm was evidence of consent. In 2012, Todd Akin (1947–2021), a Republican US representative from Missouri, aroused anger when he claimed that pregnancy rarely resulted from rape, because "if it's a legitimate rape, the female body has ways to try to shut that whole thing down."[31] The remark effectively ended Akin's political career. But it is just one example of how these older theories about reproduction continue to haunt modern policy decisions. The truism that women like sex more than men also fed into the idea that women are naturally promiscuous. Women like sex because it is fun; they do not want to get pregnant. As we will see, there was a strong connection between "loose women" and abortion.

On the Secrets of Women, which was written by a monk for his fellow monks, although it ended up reaching a wider group, primarily educated men. Many of the other texts I have cited, especially those in vernacular languages, were written, at least in part, for women. But since the Hippocratic writers, medical authors—almost exclusively male—have insisted that women can tell they are pregnant from the moment of conception. Women know they are pregnant as soon as they conceive, these authors insist, and because the fetus is most vulnerable to miscarriage in the first months of pregnancy, they should immediately take steps to prevent miscarriage. The suggestion, sometimes implicit and sometimes explicit, is that miscarriages are the result of women either being careless or deliberately trying to end their pregnancies.

HOW YOU TELL IF A WOMAN IS PREGNANT

In addition to the hydromel test described in the *Secrets of Women,* there were many ways to find out if a woman was pregnant that did not involve asking her. Although most medical authors do not explicitly advise using these techniques to trick a woman into revealing whether she has conceived, these were methods that could be performed with or without the woman's knowledge or cooperation. The hydromel test is described in many medical texts, along with similar tests that involve giving the woman something to drink and observing her reaction. For example, Guillemeau recommended: "Giue the woman Hydromell to drinke made with raine water at night when she goes to bed, or else Hony and Annisseed beaten and dissolued in water." If the woman was pregnant, in the morning she would feel pain in her abdomen. He does not suggest using subterfuge to get a woman to drink these concoctions, and in principle, there was no reason a woman could not use these methods herself. But the recommendations are written as though someone were doing them to a woman.

A handwritten family recipe book from the late seventeenth or early eighteenth century contains the hydromel test: give the woman a mixture of honey and water before she goes to bed and "if she feell Griping or paine in her belly she is with child otherwayes not." Another test from this book is to give a woman an ounce of lettuce seeds boiled in a pint of water. If this makes her vomit, she is pregnant.[32] Even in this book, which was written and used by a family that must have included women, these tests are described as things done to a woman, not techniques a woman could use to diagnose herself.

There were also multiple urine tests that could be used to determine pregnancy. In an age before indoor plumbing, where people urinated into chamber pots, and where friends, relatives, and servants regularly transported urine samples to doctors on behalf of sick people, it would not have been hard to obtain a urine sample from a woman you were living with. Again, women might have used these tests themselves, or cooperated with testers, but it would also have been possible to test a woman's urine without her knowledge. Jane Sharp said you could take a woman's urine, place a needle in it and let it sit for twenty-four hours. If at the end of the time the needle had red spots, the woman was pregnant. If the needle turned black, she was not. *Aristotle's Masterpiece* suggested a similar test, only with a "green Nettle" instead of a needle.[33] Guillemeau reported that if you take "equall quantities of the womans vrine, and of white wine" and shake them together, "if this mixture looke like the broth of Beanes, it is a signe she is with child."[34]

Of course, it is never easy to determine how many women and men in the past employed these techniques. But analysis of urine was a well-established mode of diagnosing illness, with a pedigree stretching back to Hippocrates. And there is ample evidence that people of all social and educational levels knew that changes in the color and consistency of urine indicated changes inside the body.

Techniques for determining whether a woman was pregnant can be found in handwritten collections of recipes from the sixteenth and seventeenth centuries.[35] A recipe book associated with the family of the chemist Robert Boyle (1627–1691) has the following test: "To know if a woman be with childe or noe," you should take the first urine she makes upon waking, boil it and add salt and white wine vinegar, let it cool, place it in a clear glass flask, and let it stand until the next morning. You should see sediment in the bottom of the flask. If the sediment is white, the woman is pregnant. If it is red, she is not.[36] Another recipe collection suggests placing "a new laid egg" in a woman's urine and leaving it for a day. If she was pregnant, the egg would have "white scum" on it.[37] The simplest urine test I have seen comes from a seventeenth-century manuscript recipe collection attributed to Thomas Sheppey: "To know if a woman be with Child: one way is, if you can see your hand perfectly in her water, as it stands in the Urinall."[38] Again, there is no reason women could not use these tests to analyze their own urine, but they are always written as though someone is doing the test to the woman, not as though she is doing it herself.

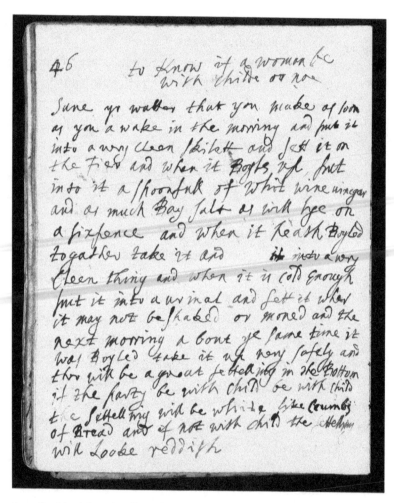

A method to determine if a woman is pregnant, from a manuscript recipe book, c. 1675–1710, belonging to Robert Boyle's family. Wellcome Collection, London, MS 1340, fol. 16v.

AVOIDING MISCARRIAGE

Premodern medical authors agreed that women experience sensations after intercourse—shivering, cold, pain, vaginal dryness—that alert them to the fact that they are pregnant. They also agreed that early detection of pregnancy was critical because the embryo was most vulnerable to miscarriage very early in pregnancy. They knew or at least suspected that a significant number of embryos were miscarried within a month or two of conception.

Soranus thought that very early in pregnancy miscarriage could be caused by strong emotions, vigorous exercise, lifting heavy objects, jumping up and down, and even coughing or sneezing. So great was the danger of miscarriage in the first few days after conception that he recommended a woman stay in bed for one or two days after conception, something she could only do if she recognized the signs of conception immediately.[39] Jacques Guillemeau agreed that the danger of miscarriage was greatest early in pregnancy: "A woman may easily loose her burthen the first moneth, because her child (though he be but little) is not yet firmely fastned and tyed to the wombe." For the first three months of pregnancy, women needed to be especially careful to avoid excessive motion and strong emotions.[40] Jane Sharp noted, "There are abundance of causes whereby women are driven to abort, or miscarry." To prevent miscarriage, she recommended that as soon as a woman conceived, she should have "natural food moderately taken" and "avoid violent passions, as care, and anger, joy, fear, or whatsoever may too much stir the blood."[41] And the author of *Aristotle's Masterpiece* writes: "After a Woman has conceived, or has any Reason to think so, she ought to be very careful of herself, lest she should do any Thing that might hinder Nature in her Operation. For in the first two Months after Conception, Women are very subject to Miscarriage, because then the Ligaments are weak, and soon broken."[42]

Miscarriages did not occur because there was something wrong with the embryo itself, and only rarely because of something done to the pregnant woman. All miscarriages were caused by shaking the delicate embryo loose from the womb. Miscarriages came about because women got up too quickly after sex, sneezed too hard, had sex again after conceiving, went dancing, rode in a carriage, got angry, or picked up a heavy object. The list of things women could do or fail to do that would cause miscarriage was near infinite. As Lara Freidenfelds writes, "Medical texts always suggested that the miscarriage happened for a reason, not entirely as a matter of chance or because of an inherent flaw in the pregnancy itself."[43] Recall the example of the pregnant woman described by Johann Storch who was beaten unconscious by a young man and in danger of miscarrying. Storch concluded that the blows to the belly that she had sustained "did not seem of great importance." Rather, the threat to the unborn child "arose more from fright and anger than from the blows."[44] Even a miscarriage following violence against a pregnant woman could be construed as her fault.

Some authors suggested that women might take advantage of the fragility of early embryos and consciously attempt to end pregnancies by engaging in vigorous activity or taking purgative drugs. Soranus states that women who wish not to be pregnant should exercise, "leap energetically," carry heavy weights, and take purgative drugs.[45] An anonymous commentary on the *Secrets of Women* points out that "the fetus, when it is first produced from the fertilized seed is attached by ligaments that are

not firm, and it is easily expelled by a certain medicine or pur-
gation." The fetus remains only weakly attached to the womb
for the first three months, a fact that "evil women" can take advantage of by having blood let or taking "certain herbal decoctions" that will dislodge the fetus.[46]

Not only were women expected to be very careful not to
cause a miscarriage by excessive motion or emotion, but they
were also expected to take steps to stop an impending miscarriage by taking appropriate medications. The current medical
consensus is that almost nothing can be done to stop a miscarriage in the first trimester. Premodern medical authors offered
considerably more hope, but they put considerably more responsibility on women to maintain pregnancies. Many suggested concoctions a woman could start drinking as soon as she
conceived to protect the embryo in those first few months of
pregnancy when the risk of miscarriage was the highest. *Aristotle's Masterpiece* recommends that a woman drink ale infused
with sage every morning as soon as she knows she is pregnant.
If a woman experiences signs of miscarriage or if she has a history of miscarriages, she can take tansy in ale, or the juice of
tansy boiled into a syrup with sugar.[47]

Jane Sharp recommended two powders that a woman could
take if she was in danger of miscarrying. The first, which would
have been quite expensive to make, consisted of powdered red
coral, ivory shavings, mastic (a kind of resin), and nutmeg. The
other was made of roots of bistort, "Kermes berries" (cochineal,
a type of insect), plantain and purslane seeds, coriander, and
sugar. This mixture was to be taken once a day in Malaga, a
sweet fortified Spanish wine.[48] Manuscript recipe books, too,
have a wide range of remedies that women could use to prevent
miscarriages. The Boyle family book has a recipe for a drink

made of rosemary and cinnamon in milk heated "over a soft fire" and drunk "hot as you can" every day for two weeks.[49] Another seventeenth-century manuscript recipe book has a more elaborate recipe that involves, among other ingredients, sarsaparilla and guaiacum wood.[50] Cochineal, sarsaparilla, and guaiacum wood were all relatively new to Europe, imported from Mexico and South America beginning in the sixteenth century. Their presence, alongside more traditional ingredients like coriander, rosemary, and cinnamon, indicates that miscarriage remedies evolved over time. The belief that women caused their own miscarriages and that these might be prevented with the right medicines was an ancient one, but the number of remedies expanded.

Another way to prevent a miscarriage was for the pregnant woman to wear an eagle stone. An eagle stone, also known as a pregnant stone or an *aetites*, was a geode with a stone inside it. Since antiquity, these have been used as amulets by pregnant women. The stone within a stone was seen as analogous to the fetus within the mother's body and exerted a kind of sympathetic magic. If the woman wore the eagle stone around her neck, it prevented miscarriage, keeping the fetus safely inside

A method to prevent miscarriages, from a manuscript recipe book, c. 1675–1710, belonging to Robert Boyle's family. Wellcome Collection, London, MS 1340, fol. 104v (detail).

her. When she went into labor, the woman would tie the eagle stone around her thigh and it would help to draw the fetus out, making for an easier birth. Pliny described the power of eagle stones in his *Natural History*,[51] and references to their use can be found on into the nineteenth century. A ninth-century Arabic medical text by Ali ibn Sahl Rabban al-Tabari mentions a family that owned a stone that would prevent miscarriage if worn by a pregnant woman.[52] When Caterina de' Medici, daughter of Christina of Lorraine, the Grand Duchess of Tuscany, married Federico Gonzaga, the Duke of Mantua, in 1617, her mother gave her an eagle stone that she herself had used during her pregnancies.[53] While the stones were valuable enough that only the wealthy could own them, some owners loaned

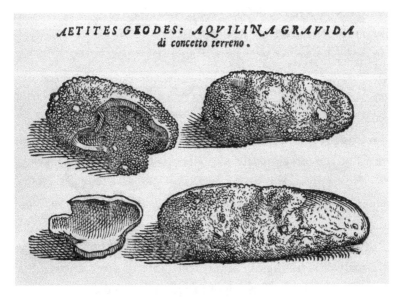

Four eagle-stone geodes, and a "pregnant eagle stone." Eagle stones, or *aetites*, were carried by pregnant women to promote childbirth from Ferranta Imperato, *Dell'historica naturale* (Naples, 1599). Wellcome Collection, London.

them out to women in need. The wealthy English landowner William Bargrave, for example, purchased an eagle stone in the 1650s and regularly loaned it out to pregnant women in his community.[54]

Looking back, we know that many women experience bleeding during pregnancy, especially early in pregnancy. Sometimes the bleeding indicates that a miscarriage is imminent, and sometimes it does not. Whether any of these remedies "worked" or not would have been a matter of luck. And yet the fact that a huge array of supposed remedies existed reinforced the notion that women should actively try to avoid miscarriage and were to blame if they failed.

THE EXPERIENCE OF PREGNANCY IN THE PRE-MODERN WORLD

The eighteenth-century German physician Johann Storch described the pregnancy of one of his patients as follows: The woman stopped menstruating in March 1723, and she believed she was pregnant. In July, she began bleeding and thought she might be miscarrying. This happened several more times before the end of the year. In February 1724, she gave birth. "Looking back," writes Barbara Duden, "we see that she had felt pregnant long before she could have been: this pregnancy had run its course between fear and hope for eleven months."[55] This case illustrates the ambiguity and uncertainty of pregnancy in the past. The robust confidence of pre-modern medical authors in the ability of women to determine pregnancy early and with certainty stands in stark contrast to the lived experience of pregnancy in the past. There may have been women in the past who claimed to know they were pregnant immediately follow-ing intercourse, but this was not the norm.

Historians who have analyzed family letters and diaries, as well as physicians' records of their consultations with female patients, paint a very different picture of pregnancy and its diagnosis in the past.[56] Pregnancy, especially in its earliest stages, was an inherently uncertain state. Another case, this time from sixteenth-century Germany, illustrates this uncertainty. The thirty-eight-year-old German noblewoman Sidonia of Braunschweig-Calenburg struggled unsuccessfully for years to get pregnant. Finally, in the late spring of 1556, she experienced the signs and symptoms of pregnancy. She told her family that she expected to give birth around Christmas. In November, she was unwell and feared that something was wrong. She sought remedies and advice from trusted female relatives to prevent miscar-riage or any harm to her unborn child. In mid-December she felt her waters break several times and was in considerable pain, but she did not go into labor as expected. Family corre-spondence reveals that it was not until early July that she and her relatives finally gave up hope that she would have a baby. Sidonia and her family believed she might be pregnant for a full year before it became obvious that she was not.[57] It is not clear whether Sidonia was never actually pregnant or whether she was pregnant and had a miscarriage. But her story illustrates that determining pregnancy in the past was much more diffi-cult than medical authors made it out to be.

For most pre-modern women and their families, the first sign of pregnancy was not a sensation of coldness after sex. The first sign was actually the same as it is today: a missed men-strual period. This is reflected in the correspondence between women and trusted family and friends. The German noblewoman

Elisabeth of Saxony (1552–1590) corresponded with her mother Anna of Saxony (1532–1585) and frequently sought her advice on reproductive matters. Soon after Elisabeth's marriage to Count Palatine John Casimir of Simmern (1543–1592) in June 1570, Anna wrote to one of the ladies at court who reported that Elisabeth had "not had her time for two months" and that there was great hope that she was pregnant. For the next fifteen years, until Anna's death in 1585, Elisabeth herself kept track of her menstrual periods and informed her mother of any irregularity that might indicate pregnancy.[58]

Marie Antoinette (1755–1793), wife of the French King Louis XVI, also corresponded regularly with her mother, the Holy Roman Empress Maria Theresa (1717–1780).[59] On April 19, 1778, she informed her mother that she had reason to hope that she was pregnant because her period was late: "I will not count on it completely until the first days of next month, time of the second cycle. Meanwhile, I believe that I have good reasons to be confident. I have never been late, on the contrary, always early. In March, I had my rules [menstrual period] on the 3rd, we are now on the 19th and there is still nothing." Her confidence was not misplaced. Her pregnancy was officially announced in May, and her first child, Marie-Thérèse Charlotte, was born on December 19, 1778.[60]

Marking the absence of menstruation was not solely a female prerogative or limited to aristocrats and royalty. Queen Elizabeth I's court astronomer John Dee (1527–1608 or 1609) kept detailed records of his wife Jane's menstrual periods as well as the times and dates of sexual intercourse.[61] On Sunday, January 1, 1660, the English civil servant Samuel Pepys wrote in his diary, "My wife, after the absence of her terms for seven weeks, gave me hopes of her being with child, but on the last day of the year she hath them again."[62] Pepys and his wife Elisabeth had been married for five years at this point and had no children. Elisabeth's delayed menses gave them reason to hope that she was finally pregnant.

A missed menstrual period was a possible sign of pregnancy, but delayed menses could have multiple causes. Barbara Duden cites numerous cases from the records of the eighteenth-century German physician Dr. Johann Storch of women whose menstruation was disrupted by fear or anger. For example, one patient was a twenty-year-old woman who was caught stealing. The fright caused her menses to stop, and they did not return for two months. During this time, the woman experienced "chills, heat, and stabbing pains," all attributed to the stopped-up blood. Another patient, a thirty-year-old woman, had a violent fit of anger that caused her menstrual flow to stop. She experienced pain around her heart and let some blood to relieve herself. Fright "caused the monthly bleeding to stagnate" and fear "[drove] the blood to the heart." Both disruptions to menstrual flow could have serious and even life-threatening consequences. In such cases, Storch prescribed remedies to restore regular menstruation.[63]

Not all women had regular menstrual periods. Some women continued to bleed during pregnancy. And some women became pregnant without ever having menstruated. The eighteenth-century French noblewoman Angélique de Mackau (1762–1800) experienced irregular menstrual patterns, meticulously described in her letters to her mother and to her husband after her marriage at the age of sixteen.[64] Her irregular menstruation complicated her efforts to determine whether she was pregnant. On several occasions, she was unsure enough that she consulted physicians to help her determine if she had conceived.

The casebooks of the English astrologer-physicians Simon Forman and Richard Napier, which document their practice between 1596 and 1634, contain thousands of records of patients of different social levels who came to the doctors with questions about reproductive matters, including whether they were pregnant.[65] These cases demonstrate the difficulties of diagnosing pregnancy. The women who consulted Foreman or Napier were confused enough about their condition to consult a physician. Some of them, like Elizabeth Borase, had stopped menstruating but were unsure if this meant they were pregnant or ill. When Borase consulted Forman, she had not menstruated in over twelve weeks, and she was experiencing pain in her lower back and abdomen, headaches, and nausea. Forman wrote: "She supposes her self with child, but I think it is not so." Instead, he diagnosed "putrefaction in her matrix [uterus]."[66] Other women had several symptoms of pregnancy but were still menstruating. When Elizabeth Leech visited Richard Napier, he noted that she had "grown bigger and bigger as a woman great with child" and that her breasts were leaking. She experienced nausea and vomiting and was "much troubled with wind & great pain in the lower part of her belly." Leech had never stopped menstruating. Napier determined that she was not pregnant, raising the troubling possibility that she had a tumor in her abdomen.[67] The Countess of Sussex consulted Napier after she had been married almost three years. She "supposes that she is now [with] child," he wrote, and "had milk in her breast." She was still menstruating every month, but her flow was "indifferent but watery." No diagnosis is recorded.[68]

A woman might also experience nausea, lack of appetite, breast tenderness, or other bodily changes. Even the authors I cited above, who claimed that women could detect conception immediately after sex, offered a whole host of other signs of pregnancy, including the one we are most familiar with, the missed menstrual period. But the missed menstrual period was just one sign of many, and not always the most important. Soon after conception, the woman's belly might be flatter than normal. She might have pain around the belly or navel and difficulty defecating. She might experience loss of appetite and nausea, or conversely a desire to eat dirt or charcoal or some other bizarre substance. Or as Jane Sharp memorably put it, a pregnant woman might have "a preternatural desire to something not fit to eat nor drink, as some women with child have longed to bite off a piece of their Husbands Buttocks."[69] The breasts swell and become tender, and the nipples change color. The veins in the breasts and under the eyes become more visible. The woman's color changes, her face becomes more flushed, and sometimes freckles develop.[70] All this suggests a tacit acknowledgment that many women missed those very earliest signs of the womb closing around the combined male and female seed. But just as today, not all women experience the same symptoms, and they could be signs of illness as well as pregnancy.

Women who had been pregnant more than once were more adept at reading the signs specific to their own bodies than were women pregnant for the first time. In a letter dated July 3, 1581, Elisabeth of Saxony informed her mother that she had not menstruated for twelve weeks and that "I feel exactly as by the other children, I vomit so very much and everything makes me feel sick, as by the other children."[71] One patient of Johann Storch had a cough and hoarse voice whenever she was pregnant. Not only did the woman herself know this as a sign that she was pregnant, but her friends and family did as well.[72] In her seventh and last pregnancy, Angélique de Mackau felt confident enough that she recognized the signs that she told her family she was pregnant when she was only two months along.[73]

The farther along the pregnancy progressed, the more certain a woman, her family, and her medical practitioners would become. "Quickening," the first time the pregnant person felt fetal movement, was a fairly sure sign of pregnancy. Many women waited until quickening to announce their pregnancies. Although Elisabeth of Saxony informed her mother Anna of Saxony when she thought she might be pregnant because her menses had stopped, she became more certain when she could report that she had felt fetal movement. After quickening, both she and her mother referred to the contents of her womb as a "fruit" or a "living fruit."[74] But quickening was not a guarantee that the pregnancy would result in a live birth. Elisabeth experienced multiple miscarriages after quickening and several stillbirths.

Further, many women missed or confused the very earliest sensations of fetal movement with gas or cramps, or simply failed to detect any motion. Johann Storch had a patient who was convinced she had a malignant "growth" in her belly because she could not feel any movement. Storch had a midwife examine her, who determined that the woman was pregnant and that the fetus was alive. Soon after, she gave birth to a healthy infant.[75] Another patient insisted that she was not pregnant even though her menses had stopped and she had a "hard and big belly." She described a cramping sensation that "moved back and forth in the belly and twitched."[76] She wanted expulsive remedies to rid herself of the "growth" and "swelling" caused by retained menses. Storch declined to help her, and she eventually gave birth. Looking back, we could say that this woman was in denial about her condition (or lying), but even married women who wanted children could be slow to distinguish the kicking of tiny feet from cramping, twitching, gas, or other bodily sensations, especially when pregnant with their first child. For example, Mary Evelyn, wife of the English diarist John Evelyn (1620–1706) was almost six months into her pregnancy before she felt fetal movement. In her second and subsequent pregnancies, she experienced quickening much earlier, an indication that she became more adept at recognizing fetal movement and distinguishing it from other bodily sensations.[77]

All of these examples point to the vast chasm between what male medical writers, like the monastic author of *On the Secrets of Women*, believed women knew about procreation and what they actually knew. Women in the past were often confused about their bodily experiences and requested help in interpreting them. The woman in total control of her fertility who could secretly terminate an unwanted pregnancy was a misogynist fantasy.

MODERN KNOWLEDGE ABOUT CONCEPTION AND MISCARRIAGE

The two-thousand-year-old belief that both women and men produced "seed" began to crumble in the eighteenth century. Spermatozoa were first seen under a microscope by Antoni van Leeuwenhoek (1632–1723) in 1677, although their role in reproduction was not immediately understood.[78] German scientist Karl Ernst von Baer discovered the mammalian egg in 1827. By the mid-nineteenth century, most doctors and scientists agreed that eggs, not seed, were released spontaneously from the ovary.

Eggs were released on a monthly cycle, not in response to sexual intercourse. In other words, ovulation and orgasm were two entirely separate phenomena. If the egg was fertilized by a sperm, the embryo would develop in the uterus. If the egg was not fertilized, menstruation followed.

Despite considerable changes in the scientific understanding of conception and early embryonic development, the notion that women can tell they are pregnant immediately after sex lingered on into the twentieth century, as we have seen. When Texas passed Senate Bill 8, the ban on abortion after a fetal heart-

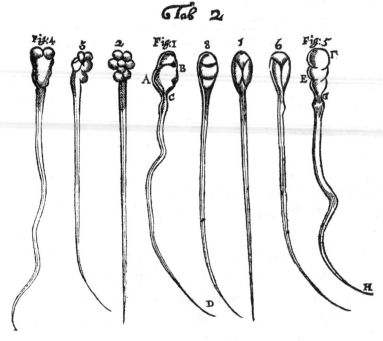

Microscopic observations of the spermatozoa of rabbit (figs. 1–4) and dog (figs. 5–8), from Anthony van Leeuwenhoek, "Observationes de natis e semine genitali animalculis," in *Philosophical Transactions* (London, 1677). Wellcome Collection, London.

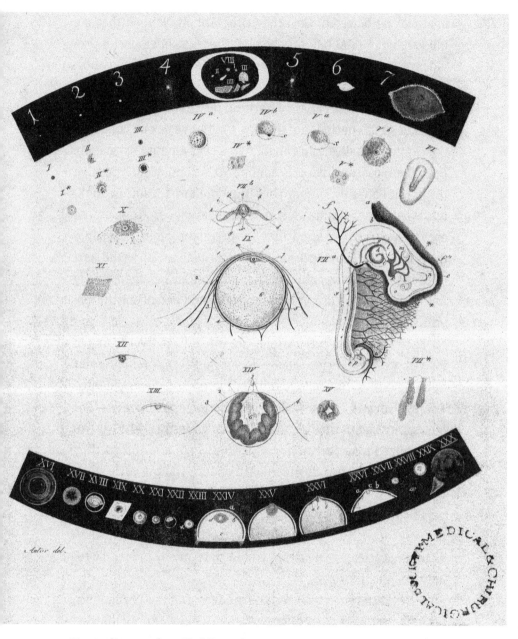

Mammalian egg, from Karl Ernst von Baer, *De ovi mammalium et hominis genesi* (1827). Wellcome Collection, London.

beat can be detected, Governor Greg Abbott claimed that the bill was not a total ban on abortion "because obviously it provides at least six weeks for a person to be able to get an abortion."[79] The ludicrousness of this remark was noted at the time. For obstetricians, pregnancy starts on the first day of a person's last menstrual period, not the day they have sex or conceive. Conception usually occurs about two weeks after menstruation. Even the most sensitive pregnancy tests will not yield a positive result until after the embryo has implanted in the uterus, about two weeks after fertilization. According to modern science, the earliest a person can know they are pregnant is four weeks into the pregnancy. Leaving aside Abbot's mistake in dating the start of pregnancy, his assumption that women know when an egg has been fertilized draws on a long outdated and deeply misogynistic strain of thought.

Each menstrual cycle, which can range from twenty-one to forty days, the ovaries release an egg, or occasionally two or more eggs, into the Fallopian tube, a process called ovulation. The egg lingers in the Fallopian tube for about twenty-four hours. During this time—and only during this time—the egg can be fertilized by a sperm. If it is not fertilized, it is absorbed by the body or expelled during menstruation, and the cycle starts again. The menstrual cycle is taken to begin on the first day of a person's menstrual period. Ovulation typically occurs about halfway through the cycle. For a person with the average twenty-eight-day cycle, menstruation would start on day one and ovulation on day fourteen.

A key difference between the modern and the pre-modern understanding of reproduction is that we now know that sex and conception are rarely simultaneous. Sperm can survive in the Fallopian tube for up to five days. It is possible to have sex on Monday, to ovulate on Thursday, and for the egg to be fertilized on Friday. In fact, people who are trying to get pregnant are advised to have sex a few days before ovulation so there are sperm waiting in the Fallopian tube for the egg. Following fertilization, the egg starts dividing into multiple cells and travels through the Fallopian tube toward the uterus. By five to six days after fertilization the embryo is at the blastocyst stage. At seven days after fertilization, the blastocyst implants in the uterus. During implantation, the embryo begins to produce human chorionic gonadotropin (hCG). This is the hormone that home pregnancy tests can detect.

In sum, an embryo implants in the uterus a full week after fertilization and up to two weeks after the sex that led to fertilization. It is at least another full week before the levels of hCG in the pregnant person's body are high enough to be detected by a home pregnancy test, although it can take longer. This would be right around the time the next menstrual period would be expected. Given this understanding of conception, it makes no sense to claim that a woman could know she was pregnant after sex, because this is almost always a few days before fertilization occurs and a few weeks before any of the physical symptoms of pregnancy, including a missed period and a positive home pregnancy test, begin to manifest themselves.

Along with a changed understanding of the process of ovulation, fertilization, and implantation, understandings of miscarriages have changed as well. Pre-modern texts describe miscarriage as "common" and the risk as highest during the earliest months of pregnancy. Today we know that a significant percentage of embryos do not implant in the uterus. They are resorbed by the body or expelled during the next menstrual period. This type of very early miscarriage is indistinguishable from a regular menstrual period. Because the embryo never implants, the pregnant person's body never produces hCG and there will be no positive pregnancy test.

Estimates of how many embryos are lost before implantation range from 10 to 40 percent.[80] After implantation, somewhere between 10 and 20 percent of pregnancies end in miscarriage, almost all within the first three months. Combining miscarriages pre- and post-implantation, about a quarter of all pregnancies end in miscarriage.[81] What these figures mean is that pregnancy loss is a normal and common part of reproductive life. A high percentage of women who have tried to get pregnant, or have gotten pregnant unexpectedly, have had at least one miscarriage. In one study of over fifty thousand women, 43 percent reported having had at least one first-trimester miscarriage.[82] Many miscarriages, especially when they occur before implantation, go unrecognized.

Now we not only know how common miscarriages are, we also have a better understanding of what causes them. Although obstetricians are not yet able to diagnose the cause of each miscarriage, and most people who miscarry will never know what triggered their specific miscarriage, we do know that most early pregnancy loss is caused by chromosomal abnormalities in the embryo. We also know that the actions pre-modern medical writers believed caused miscarriage—dancing, jumping, running, riding a carriage along a bumpy road, getting angry, being frightened, and having sex—do not cause miscarriage. But the idea that exercise, work, stress, and sex can cause pregnancy loss still has a tight hold on the popular imagination.

The website of the American College of Obstetricians and Gynecologists states:

> In almost every case, miscarriage is not a woman's fault.
> This is important to understand. Miscarriage usually is a
> random event. Working, exercising, stress, arguments, [or]
> having sex...do not cause miscarriage....Some women
> who have had a miscarriage believe that it was caused by
> a recent fall, blow, fright, or stress. In most cases, this is
> not true. It may simply be that these things happened to
> occur around the same time and are fresh in the
> memory.[83]

The fact that so many medical websites like this one contain a
list of things that do *not* cause miscarriages, and that these lists
are all full of things that pre-modern medical texts stated caused
miscarriage, is an indication of how these ideas have survived
into the twenty-first century.

Surveys conducted in the early twenty-first century show
that many Americans continue to hold long-outdated beliefs
about the causes of miscarriage. In 2015 the journal *Obstetrics
and Gynecology* published "A National Survey on Public Perceptions of Miscarriage." Researchers compiled a list of sixteen possible causes of miscarriage. For each item, participants were
asked whether they agreed that it was a cause of miscarriage,
disagreed, or were unsure. Almost all participants correctly
agreed that "genetic abnormalities of the fetus" are a cause of
miscarriage. But a majority also incorrectly agreed that stress
and lifting heavy objects could cause miscarriage, 21 percent of
respondents believed that getting into an argument could cause
a miscarriage, and 23 percent believed not wanting to be pregnant could cause a miscarriage. While it is possible that stress
contributes to miscarriage, the data on this is unclear. There is

no evidence that lifting heavy objects, arguing, or not wanting to be pregnant causes miscarriages.

Further, "Twenty-two percent of participants incorrectly believed that lifestyle choices, such as drug, alcohol, or tobacco use during pregnancy, are the single most common cause of miscarriage, more common than genetic or medical causes. Men were 2.6 times more likely to believe this than women."[84] A more recent study published in 2020 surveyed attitudes toward pregnancy loss in men, trans/masculine, and nonbinary people. This was a smaller-scale study, with fifty-one participants, but the results were similar. One of the study participants blamed his miscarriage on not "eating right." Another attributed his pregnancy loss to "the stress of illness and a death in the family."[85]

These studies document the ongoing salience of pre-modern understandings of miscarriage, but they do not address the source of these beliefs. Another study of attitudes toward miscarriage from 2005 categorizes these beliefs as "folkloric" and "old wives' tales."[86] The author describes these as "beliefs that circulate among lay members of the community." Although he concedes that "some have some historical root in mainstream medicine," he asserts that "they have been abandoned by the medical community as pregnancy physiology has become better understood." In fact, every single one of these beliefs, as we have seen, has a long history in medical texts. But his contention is that physicians are not disseminating these beliefs, women themselves are "because they fill a need to rationalize events that are largely beyond a woman's control."[87] On the surface, it might seem that he is correct. After all, as I pointed out, many websites by reputable medical providers and organizations clearly state that miscarriages are not caused by exercise, stress, work, sex, anger, or fright. And yet medical practitioners are complicit in spreading misinformation about miscarriages and in blaming women for pregnancy loss.

In the conclusion to her study of the history of miscarriage in America, Lara Freidenfelds criticizes public health messages that lead pregnant people to believe that if they just follow all their doctor's advice, eat right, and avoid alcohol and caffeine, then they will have a healthy child. The reality is that many people will do everything "right" and still end up miscarrying. Giving people who could become pregnant more honest information about the frequency of miscarriage would, in her view, alleviate the feelings of guilt that so frequently accompany miscarriages. But she notes: "At my talks for medical and public health professionals, some have suggested that telling women the truth about the commonness of early pregnancy loss would lead them to be less careful about taking care of their pregnancies. Better, they say, to encourage women to bond with their early pregnancies so that the pregnancies that do succeed will be healthier."[88] As Freidenfelds points out, this approach does nothing to help women who lack access to medical care, healthy food, clean water, and other resources necessary to maintain a healthy pregnancy, or who struggle with addiction, or who are in abusive relationships. And it leads pregnant people to blame themselves for miscarriages.

But doctors and other medical professionals are more directly implicated in the widespread tendency to blame women for miscarriages. Women like Poolaw who are prosecuted for their miscarriages come to the attention of prosecutors only because their medical providers report them to the police. For example, Lizelle Herrera, a twenty-six-year-old Texas woman, was arrested in April 2022 for allegedly causing the "death of an individual by self-induced abortion," even though self-induced abortion is not actually a crime in Texas.[89] Herrera, like Poolaw, ended up in jail because medical personnel at the hospital where she sought care called the police. Speaking about the case, Rockie Gonzalez, founder of the Frontera Fund, an organization that provides financial support to people seeking abortions, said: "Low income people of color cannot walk into a hospital safely and know that they will be able to be honest with their medical providers and give them information that might save their life because they might go to jail."[90]

In her book on racism and infant mortality, Monica Casper addresses the tendency to blame women, especially Black women, for infant death. Casper writes: "Lodging blame with mothers is a misogynistic sleight of hand that draws the eye away from structural causes of infant mortality, such as poverty and racism. Because if women are to blame, then we need not worry about unequal access to healthcare, violence, environmental toxins, food deserts, or the many other factors that contribute to high rates of infant—and maternal—death."[91] Her point can be extended to miscarriage. Blaming women, like Brittney Poolaw, for their miscarriages is a way of evading questions about the ways poverty and racism increase the risk of miscarriage.

Comanche County, where Poolaw lived, has at least thirty active fracking sites.[92] Fracking, as I pointed out in the last chapter, is known to raise rates of miscarriage in adjacent areas.[93] What if, instead of asking about her drug use, doctors, police, and the prosecutor had asked about her proximity to these sites? Or investigated the quality of the drinking water available to her? What if, instead of looking for reasons to blame her, they took a hard look at the obstacles to a healthy pregnancy facing Poolaw? And what if, rather than blaming her for failing to overcome these obstacles, they worked to provide healthier, safer living conditions for her and for other Oklahoma women? "It is just so much *easier* to blame women," writes Casper. "Women are potentially malleable; social structures much less so."[94]

What would it look like to place the blame for miscarriages on the social structures that prevent women from having healthy pregnancies? To answer that, I conclude with the story of Virginia mother Sharanda Taylor. In February 2018, Taylor addressed the Richmond City Council and described the living conditions she and her children were forced to endure in the city's public housing. Their apartment had no heat and was infested with mice. Taylor revealed that she had suffered a miscarriage and blamed her pregnancy loss on the substandard housing and the stress it caused her. She drove the point home by showing the council members a plastic cup containing her miscarried fetus. "This is a baby," Taylor said, "my embryo that I can no longer carry." Through tears Taylor added, "I sit here watching people hold their babies in the back while I hold mine in a cup."[95]

Given the frequency of miscarriages, Taylor might have lost her baby even if she had clean, safe housing, healthy food, and top-quality medical care. Wealth and privilege did not protect Chan, Underwood, and Markle from pregnancy loss. And yet in drawing attention to the material conditions of her life, Taylor highlights that poverty, racism, and environmental hazards increase the risk of miscarriage. Taylor deserved the opportunity to give her unborn child the best odds of survival. She, unlike the prosecutor and jury that put Brittney Poolaw in jail, has put the blame for her miscarriage where it belongs.

5

ABORTION AND THE FETUS

I have traced the long history, going back to the ancient world, of treating mother and fetus as two distinct entities. I have discussed the ways that accounts of embryonic and fetal development have been kept separate from accounts of pregnancy and pointed out that the former has commanded far more attention than the latter. And I have examined the historical roots of the belief that the relationship between the pregnant person and the fetus is antagonistic and that the fetus requires protection from its mother. I pointed to the relevance of this history to our current debates about abortion. Most of the history that I have recounted is unfamiliar except to those scholars who specialize in the history of pregnancy and childbirth.

In what follows, I turn to the history of abortion itself, exploring some of its medical, legal, and moral dimensions. Unlike the history in the first four chapters, much of the material in this chapter will be at least somewhat familiar. The history of abortion is well-trodden territory. Even if you are not a specialist in ancient gynecology, you might have heard that the Hippocratic oath prohibits abortion. Even if you are not a scholar of early Christianity, you might know that the church father Saint Augustine condemned abortion. And there are several good books and many excellent articles on the history of abortion in the United States.[1] This history is familiar because it is frequently invoked in debates about abortion. Both opponents and supporters of legal abortion have claimed that their position has both ancient precedent and deep historical roots.

In the landmark *Roe v. Wade* decision of 1973 that legalized abortion in the United States, Chief Justice Harry Blackmun, author of the majority opinion, began with a medical and legal history of abortion. Blackmun intended to demonstrate that the criminalization of abortion was a relatively new phenomenon, not an age-old principle. English common law made a distinction between an abortion before "quickening" and after. Quickening was "the first recognizable movement of the fetus in utero" and a sign that the fetus had developed far enough to have an independent life. "It is undisputed," he wrote, "that at common law, abortion performed before 'quickening' . . . was not an indictable offense." And in the United States, "the law in effect in all but a few States until mid-nineteenth century was the pre-existing English common law." Thus, at the time of the adoption of the US Constitution, abortion before quickening was legal and accepted.

Establishing the legal situation at the time of the writing and acceptance of the Constitution had obvious bearing on the question of whether abortion could be considered a constitutional right. But Blackmun traced the roots of abortion back much further, to the ancient Greeks and Romans. In the ancient world, abortion was practiced "without scruple," according to Blackmun. The philosophers Aristotle and Plato explicitly condoned abortion, as did the Roman physician Galen. To the extent that abortion was ever regarded as a crime in the ancient world, it was because it was a violation of the "father's right to his offspring."[2]

Forty-nine years later, in the *Dobbs v. Jackson Women's Health Organization* decision of 2022 that overturned *Roe v. Wade*, Justice Samuel Alito offered a very different account of the history of abortion. The history presented in the *Roe* decision ranged, he asserted, "from the constitutionally irrelevant (e.g., its discussion of abortion in antiquity) to the plainly incorrect (e.g., its assertion that abortion was probably never a crime under the common law)." Instead of Blackmun's broad sweep of history beginning in the ancient world, Alito confined himself to the writings of four "eminent common-law authorities," English judges and legal scholars ranging from the thirteenth to the eighteenth century. These were Henry of Bracton (c. 1210–1268), author of *On the Laws and Customs of England*; Edward Coke (1552–1634), author of *Institutes of the Lawes of England*; Matthew Hale (1609–1676), author of *The History of the Pleas of the Crown*; and William Blackstone (1723–1780), author of *Commentaries on the Laws of England*. All four of these authorities, he claimed, "wrote that a post-quickening abortion was a crime," and Hale and Blackstone held that "even a pre-quickening abortion was unlawful." "The inescapable conclusion," Alito wrote, "is that a right to abortion is not deeply rooted in the Nation's history and traditions. On the contrary, an unbroken tradition of prohibiting abortion on pain of criminal punishment persisted from the earliest days of the common law until 1973."[3]

The differences in Blackmun's and Alito's histories of abortion highlight the fact that sources for writing a history of abortion are abundant. We have medical books that describe methods of inducing abortion as well as discussions of when abortion is medically necessary. We have religious and philosophical writing on the morality of abortion. We have laws and records of criminal prosecutions for abortion. You can construct different stories depending on which sources you use and how you interpret those sources. This does not mean all possible stories are equally accurate, but it does mean anyone can find historical precedent for their position on abortion. Blackmun, for example, also cited Bracton, Coke, and Blackstone, but he used these authors to demonstrate that common law made a distinction between the abortion of a fetus before and after quickening, and he highlighted the disagreements between these authors to argue that it was "doubtful that abortion was ever firmly established as a common-law crime even with respect to the destruction of a quick fetus."[4]

One striking similarity between the pro-life history of abortion traced by Alito and the pro-choice history outlined by Blackmun is that all the sources they use are by men. Despite the plethora of opinions on abortion over the centuries, historians lack what Tara Mulder drily refers to as "a uterus-carrying perspective on the matter."[5] This has serious ramifications for the kinds of history we can trace, as law professor Jill Elaine Hasday points out in her critique of Alito's argument: "Alito relies on sources such as [Matthew] Hale without acknowledging their entanglement with legalized male supremacy." Matthew Hale sentenced women to death for witchcraft, argued that women generally lied about rape, and asserted that there was no such thing as marital rape because husbands were in control of their wives' bodies. None of the four common-law authorities cited by Alito believed women should have anything remotely close to equal rights with men.[6] Failing to find precedent or justification for a right to abortion in these authors' books is like failing to find the proverbial snowball in hell. I cannot hope to remedy the imbalance in the source material. But I do intend to dwell on the absence of "a uterus-carrying perspective" and its implications for our understanding of the histories of abortion.

My account of the history of abortion is structured around the stories of three women and their abortions: a Greek slave, an Irish princess, and a midwestern mother. In each case, their stories were originally told by men. Indeed, in each case, a man is the hero of the story, "rescuing" a woman whose thoughts, emotions, desires, and intentions are conspicuously absent from the story. I cannot claim to know what the women in these stories thought or felt, but in each case, I interrogate *why* the woman's perspective was omitted from the narrative. I use each story to explore different facets of the history of abortion. My aim is not to produce a comprehensive history of abortion from ancient times to the present. Rather, I want to draw attention to how much of the history of abortion, especially before the nineteenth century, relies on sources written by men about women, and by men who had generally negative views of women's bodies and women's minds. Our reliance on these sources has shaped—and distorted—what we think we know about abortion in the past.

The story of the Greek slave girl shows that long before the modern concepts of fetal personhood and fetal rights emerged, the fetus was viewed as an entity distinct from its mother, and an object that did not belong to its mother. Mothers were just caretakers of fetuses, and poor caretakers at that. Many men objected to abortion on grounds that the fetus was not the mother's to dispose of and claimed that women only sought abortions to cover up sexual misbehavior and to avoid the physical demands of pregnancy and childbirth. For the pre-modern period, we have virtually no accounts of abortions by women that would counter this narrative.

I use the story of the Irish princess to examine the complex and varying stance on abortion within the history of Christianity. Her story demonstrates that medieval Christians could in certain circumstances see abortion as holy rather than sinful. There is ample evidence that Christians today who support abortion rights are every bit as traditional as those who oppose abortion. Finally, I use the story of the midwestern mother to explore the different methods for inducing abortion in the past. These methods remain remarkably consistent from the ancient period up until the early twentieth century. Her story also points to the ways that abortion care in the past was closely connected to other forms of obstetrical and gynecological care, including contraception, easing labor pain, miscarriage care, and menstrual regulation. Her case illustrates that the importance of menstrual regularity opened an ambiguous space where early abortions might be conducted discreetly, arouse little suspicion, and leave no trace.

THE GREEK SLAVE

The story of the Greek slave appears at the beginning of the Hippocratic text *Nature of the Child* and is narrated by a physician.

A female relative of mine once owned a very valuable singing girl who had relations with men, but who was not to become pregnant lest she lose her value. The singing girl had heard what women say to one another, that when a woman is about to conceive, the seed does not run out of her, but remains inside. She understood what she heard and always paid attention, and when she one time noticed that the seed did not run out of her, she told her mistress, and the case came to me. When I heard (sc. what had happened), I told her to spring up and down so as to kick her heels against her buttocks, and when she had sprung for the seventh time, the seed ran out on to the ground with a noise, and the girl on seeing it gazed at it and was amazed.[7]

Bearing in mind that the story is told by a physician, and that it serves to emphasize his knowledge of the female body and of fetal development, we should not take this as a straightforward or representative account of how abortions were typically performed in ancient Greece. It is likely that women more commonly turned to other women for help with this and other reproductive matters. It suggests that male physicians were interested in and knowledgeable about pregnancy and that they could be called on to perform abortions. The six-day-old embryo, as described by the physician, does not have a recognizably human form, so this story is consistent with a view that a very young embryo does not have a human soul, although there is no comment on whether an abortion at a later stage of pregnancy would or would not be acceptable.

For me, the most striking thing about this story is that it is not "pro-choice." This is not a story about a woman choosing to end an unwanted pregnancy. Quite the reverse, the girl in this story has no reproductive or bodily autonomy at all. She is used by her mistress as a sex worker, and pregnancy would diminish her economic value. Her views on the abortion are not recorded, because they were not relevant to either her mistress or the physician. The story is set in a world in which some people had the right to procreate and others did not. It is not a story about a married woman who has decided she does not want to be pregnant.

In the ancient Greek world, married women were expected to bear and raise children, and children were under the legal and moral authority of their fathers. Konstantinos Kapparis comments that the sexual activity of "females designated to become mothers of legitimate heirs and future citizens" was tightly restricted to ensure "the legitimacy of the offspring."[8] We might expect a relaxed attitude toward abortion in a society that condoned the exposure of unwanted infants. But children, including fetuses, belonged to their fathers. The decision about whether to accept a newborn into the family or abandon it was the father's.[9] As Tara Mulder notes, in the ancient Roman world, condemnations of abortion "rest not, as they do today, on the notion that a fetus is a person, but on the notion that a fetus belongs to its father and to the state."[10] In his "Speech in Defense of Aulus Cluentius Habitus," the Roman philosopher, politician, and orator Marcus Tullius Cicero (106–43 BCE) recalled the case of a woman condemned to death for having an abortion. Death was an appropriate punishment, he commented, not because this woman had killed another human being, but because "she had cheated the father of his hopes, his name of continuity, his family of its support, his house of an heir, and the Republic of a citizen-to-be."[11]

According to Mulder, Roman writers frequently condemned abortion and associated the practice with female vanity and promiscuity.[12] Pliny the Elder (23/24–79) wrote that "males have devised every out-of-the-way form of sexual indulgence, crimes against nature, but the females have invented abortion."[13] The historian Tacitus (c. 56–c. 120) records that the emperor Nero's (37–68) wife Octavia was accused of having an abortion to hide her adulterous affair.[14] In his *Attic Nights*, Aulus Gellius (second century CE) decries women, "who strive by evil devices to cause abortion of the fetus itself which they have conceived, in order that their beauty may not be spoiled by the weight of the burden they bear and by the labour of parturition."[15] The second-century CE satirist Juvenal claims, in a virulently misogynistic poem, that rich women refuse to undergo the hardships of pregnancy and childbirth and instead avail themselves of "the skills and drugs of the woman who manufactures sterility and takes contracts to kill humans inside the belly."[16] As this last example makes clear, the Romans sometimes equated abortion with the killing of a human being,[17] although Roman law did not treat abortion as equivalent to homicide. For centuries, male writers offered these same condemnations of women who sought to end their pregnancies: they were vain, self-indulgent, immoral, and promiscuous.

Distrust of women also comes across in the *Gynecology* of the Roman physician Soranus. It is not acceptable, he writes, to help a woman "to destroy the embryo because of adultery or out of consideration for youthful beauty." But Soranus grants that there are cases in which it would be dangerous for a woman to continue a pregnancy, for example, "if the uterus is small and not capable of accommodating the complete development" of the fetus. He does not suggest the use of either contraceptives or abortifacients to limit family size or for any other reason than risk to the life of the mother. In such cases, it is safer to avoid conception with the use of contraceptives than to resort to abortion, and he lists multiple substances to put in or around the vagina to prevent pregnancy. But for cases where it is medically necessary to end a pregnancy, he provides recipes for compounds to be taken orally or to be administered as vaginal suppositories.[18]

The philosopher Aristotle offers yet another window into ancient attitudes toward abortion. Aristotle advocated abortion as a means of maintaining a healthy population and of keeping the size of the population at a level proportionate to resources. In his *Politics*, Aristotle proposes that in an ideal society, the number of children born will be proportional to the resources available. In other words, population growth should be carefully monitored so as not to exceed the food supply. Accordingly, leaders should make laws setting limits on who can marry, at what ages, and how many children they can have. To remove excess children, newborns can be exposed, or women can be encouraged (or forced) to have abortions. If abortion is used to control population size, it must be done "before [the fetus] has developed sensation and life; for the line between lawful and unlawful abortion will be marked by the fact of having sensation and being alive."[19] For Aristotle, abortion and infanticide are both legitimate measures to maintain the health and vigor of a population. As in the Hippocratic story of the slave, there is no sense that the needs or desires of pregnant women or mothers of newborns are relevant.

In sum, the ancient Greeks and Romans were more ambivalent about abortion than Blackmun's assertion that they practiced abortion "without scruple" implied. They thought of the fetus as distinct from its mother, but that does not mean they thought of it as a person, as modern opponents of abortion do. Their objection to abortion was that the fetus did not belong to the mother, and she should not be the one to decide its fate.[20]

This is consistent with their understanding of conception and fetal development. Greco-Roman theories of generation attributed the active role in making a baby to the father. The mother's role was passive. She provided warmth and food for the offspring. Like a baker putting a bun in the oven to bake, the father did the real formative, creative work. And the resulting fetus belonged to him.

Arguments that abortion is wrong because the fetus is not the property of the pregnant woman and thus not hers to dispose of as she wishes would reemerge with a vengeance in the diatribes of eighteenth- and nineteenth-century slaveowners. The notion of the fetus as property, and property that does not belong to the pregnant woman, is nowhere clearer than in the reproductive histories of enslaved Black people. As Dorothy Roberts writes, "Slaveowners perceived the Black fetus as a separate entity that would produce future profits or that could be parceled out to another owner before its birth."[21]

Throughout the eighteenth and nineteenth centuries, the stereotype of the malicious and promiscuous Black woman who killed her own children, both those in the womb and those already born, circulated widely across the slave societies of the Caribbean and the Americas. Slave midwives, too, were frequently accused of helping women end their pregnancies or dispose of unwanted newborns.[22] Rather than attributing low birth rates and excessive infant deaths to the conditions of slavery—grueling physical labor, brutal physical punishments, poor-quality nutrition, and unhygienic living conditions—slaveowners frequently accused Black women of using contraceptives, inducing abortions, and even killing their babies.[23] A French pro-slavery pamphlet published in 1790 accused enslaved Black women of "destroy[ing] their own fruit" by inducing abortions and murdering their newborns when this failed. They did this, or so the pamphlet claimed, because having to take care of children would interfere with their sex lives.[24] In the minds of slaveowners, abortion and infanticide were closely related crimes. They were crimes, not because a person was being killed when an enslaved woman had an abortion, or even when a newborn was murdered, but because the slaveowner's property was being destroyed.

The fact that abortion was practiced in the ancient world—along with contraception and infanticide—does not mean that women in the past had as much or more reproductive autonomy than they do today. There was opposition to abortion long before the concept of fetal personhood was first articulated. The ancients did not need to see the fetus as a person, or to believe that every human being was worthy of life, to condemn abortion. Whether we read Roman writers railing against adulterous wives or nineteenth-century slaveowners fulminating about treacherous Black mothers, the wickedness of women is a constant theme in opposition to abortion. This theme will carry over into Christian opposition to abortion and continues to inform pro-life arguments in the present.

The need to control women's sexual and reproductive activities runs through much ancient (and modern) opposition to abortion. To return to the story of the Greek slave girl, notice that the physician can terminate her pregnancy only because the girl revealed to her mistress that she was pregnant. No one would have known that she was six days pregnant without her testimony. Of course, the pregnancy would have become apparent eventually. But most abortions, then as now, took place very early in pregnancy. Aside from the belief that a very young embryo did not yet have a human soul, it was widely agreed that it was easiest and safest to terminate a pregnancy soon after conception. Later-term abortions were less likely to be successful and more likely to result in the death of the pregnant person. This means that most abortions took place before anyone except the woman and her trusted confidants were aware of the pregnancy. Most abortions would have taken place quietly and privately. As we will see, the substances used to induce abortions were not hard to obtain, and most were used in a variety of medicines, so their purchase or possession would not arouse suspicion. Hence the tremendous anxiety of male writers convinced that women were up to no good. Unless a woman reported her pregnancy to an authority figure—husband, physician, slaveowner—how could they hope to control her?

THE IRISH PRINCESS

Once upon a time (about 500 CE), there was an Irish princess named Bruinnech, who was both beautiful and virtuous. She entered the monastery of Ciarán of Saigir and vowed a life of perpetual virginity. But a wicked king, Dímma, saw her and succumbed to lust and greed. He kidnapped and raped Bruinnech. By the time Ciarán rescued her and returned her to his monastery, she was pregnant. Ciarán "pressed down on her womb with the sign of the cross and forced her womb to be emptied."[25] After her ordeal, Bruinnech resumed her life in the monastery.

The tale of Bruinnech's abortion is part of an account of the life and miracles of Saint Ciarán. Ciarán is one of four early (fifth- and sixth-century) Irish saints who performed miraculous abortions on women whose fetuses were the product of rape, incest, or fornication. Áed mac Bricc blessed the womb of a nun who had secretly had sex and gotten pregnant. Cainnech of Aghaboe similarly blessed the womb of an unmarried pregnant woman. In both cases, the "blessing" caused the unborn child to vanish. One female saint, Brigid of Kildare, is also credited with a miraculous abortion. In these three cases, the names of the women are not even mentioned in the saints' biographies. In no case does the woman in the story directly ask the saint to end her pregnancy. The decision appears to be the saint's alone. As historian Maeve Callan describes the story of Bruinnech, her "body was the battlefield for a war waged between religious and secular male authority." Dímma stole her away from Ciarán, "and she subsequently seems little more than the site of one man's effacement of another's virility."[26] Like the Greek slave girl, the Irish princess had no choice, in the circumstances of her pregnancy or in its termination. These "holy abortions," as Callan has dubbed them, were unusual, but they remind us that there was (and is) a wide range of possible views on the morality of abortion among Christians.[27]

Saint-induced abortions were, of course, not the only type of abortion available in early medieval Ireland. Women might also turn to someone with knowledge of "herbs" or "magic." Irish penitentials—that is, texts that list sins and the appropriate penance for each—of this period include abortion. Significantly, abortion was a relatively minor sin. Further, "whenever the Irish penitentials identified the gender of those with such abilities, the abortionists were always female."[28] If a saint performed an abortion, it was a miracle; if a female medical practitioner gave a woman some herbs to induce abortion, this was a sin.

None of this suggests a worldview where women have bodily autonomy and control of their reproductive lives. But neither does it suggest a worldview where abortion is an unqualified evil. As Callan and other scholars of early Christianity have argued, it is simply not the case that the Catholic Church ever had one unequivocal stance on abortion. A month before Irish citizens voted to repeal their constitution's eighth amendment, which banned almost all abortions, Callan wrote, "Those who support legal and safe abortion might better reflect a 'medieval' Irish Catholic attitude than those who oppose it."[29] And after Texas S.B. 8, the Texas Heartbeat Act, went into effect in September 2021, Luis Josué Salés asserted that "Christians who support women's reproductive rights are also following the historical precedent of their religious tradition."[30] I chose Bruinnech's story because "holy" and "miraculous" and abortion are about the last words modern readers expect to see together.

In the modern world, opposition to abortion is religious, and near exclusively Christian, although anti-abortion groups and individuals frequently insist that secular science is on their side. Both Catholic and Protestant opponents of abortion often claim that Christians have always opposed abortion and have always believed that human life begins at conception. The official position of the Catholic Church, for example, is that they have *always* believed and taught that life begins at conception and that abortion at all stages of pregnancy is sinful. The catechism of the Catholic Church states: "Since the first century the Church has affirmed the moral evil of every procured abortion. This teaching *has not changed and remains unchangeable*. Direct abortion, that is to say, abortion willed either as an end or a means, is gravely contrary to the moral law." The United States Conference of Catholic Bishops has produced a "fact sheet" on "Respect for Unborn Human Life: The Church's Constant Teaching." "From earliest times," the USCCB asserts, "Christians sharply distinguished themselves from surrounding pagan cultures by rejecting abortion and infanticide." As evidence, the fact sheet references the *Didache* (Teaching of the Twelve Apostles) and the *Letter of Barnabas*, two documents from the first and second centuries of the Church that both condemn abortion, as well as "early regional and particular Church councils." The church father Augustine of Hippo condemned abortion, as did the great medieval theologian Thomas Aquinas. In 1869 Pope Pius IX declared that abortion *at all stages* was a mortal sin, carrying the penalty of automatic excommunication. This officially removed the "obsolete distinction" between abortion before and after "ensoulment." This, the bishops maintain, was not a new policy but merely the natural extension of the existing position that abortion was "gravely wrong at every stage."[31]

Evangelical Protestant anti-abortion groups make similar claims. The organization Abolish Human Abortion states on its website that early Christians "consistently set themselves in bold opposition to their culture's widespread practices of bloodsport, infanticide, child-abandonment, and abortion."[32] But as we have seen, the ancient Greeks and Romans were at best reluctant supporters of abortion. Although they acknowledged that it was sometimes necessary to preserve a woman's health or life, they thought the decision to terminate a pregnancy rightfully belonged to the father, or sometimes the state (as in Aristotle's scheme for population control) or the slaveowner. How much did early Christian attitudes toward abortion really differ from those of their pagan neighbors?

Attitudes toward abortion in the early church were part of a new, distinctively Christian understanding of sexuality and sexual morality. Following Augustine, theologians and preachers in the early centuries of Christianity asserted that the sole purpose of sex was procreation. Only married people should have sexual intercourse, and they should only engage in sexual acts that might lead to conception. Contraception was deeply wrong because it subverted the natural, God-given purpose of sex. Or put another way, it perverted sex by turning it into something done purely for pleasure. Abortion was wrong for the same reason. It detached sex from procreation. The equation of contraception and early abortion was strengthened by the fact that frequently the same herbs were used for both, as we shall see.

Because early Christians adopted the mainstream Greek view of fetal development that held that ensoulment happened sometime after conception, they did not equate early abortions with homicide. The notion that abortion at all stages of pregnancy is tantamount to murder is one that developed much later in the history of Christianity. This is not to say that no theologian in the early centuries of the Christian churches adopted the Aristotelian view that ensoulment and conception were simultaneous. Some did. But this was never the only or even the majority view on abortion.

Medieval Christian condemnations of abortion often sound remarkably like ancient pagan condemnations in that they harp on the sexual sins and treachery of women.[33] The anonymous thirteenth-century monk who wrote *On the Secrets of Women* complained that "evil women" abort their fetuses by having blood drawn or taking herbal decoctions. Most physicians believed that letting blood early in pregnancy was dangerous and could cause a miscarriage. Allegedly, some women took advantage of this to end unwanted pregnancies.[34] Similarly, it was widely believed that early in pregnancy, women should avoid moving around too vigorously or lifting heavy objects because these actions could shake the fetus loose from the womb and cause miscarriage. This same author complained that "some evil women who are aware of this and counsel young girls who have become pregnant and wish to hide their sin that they should jump around, run, walk, and briskly move about in order to corrupt the fetus."[35] Given that the writer was a monk writing for monks, we may question how much personal experience he had with pregnant women. By the thirteenth century, the caricature of women who have abortions "to hide their sin" was very old indeed.

However, unlike ancient pagan authors, Christians sometimes held men to the same standards of sexual purity as women. The late fourth-century bishop John Chrysostom taught that abortion was sinful but refused to put all the blame on the pregnant woman. He declared that if a man got a sex worker pregnant and she had an abortion, then he was more to blame for the abortion than she was. The sex worker depended for her livelihood on "being agreeable and an object of longing to her lovers," while her client had no such excuse. "For even if the daring deed be hers," Chrysostom said, "yet the causing of it is yours."[36]

The notion that sexual intercourse was solely for procreation put Christianity at odds with the surrounding pagan cultures in its early centuries, but it also put it at odds with Jewish and Muslim understandings of sexuality, as well as with contemporary medical theory, which held that regular sex was necessary for health, especially for women. Many medical authors, both among the ancient Greeks and Romans and among medieval Islamic physicians, taught that sex was essential to a woman's health. While a Catholic theologian might argue that a woman who should not get pregnant because, for example, her uterus was too small for a fetus to develop normally, should simply not have sex, a medical author might argue that sex was necessary for her health and that she should use contraceptives and, if these failed, abortifacients. This contradiction remained largely unresolved throughout the medieval and early modern periods.[37]

An example of this tension can be found in the work of the translator Constantine the African (d. c. 1099 CE).[38] Originally a Muslim merchant from Tunis in North Africa, he traveled to southern Italy in the 1060s or 1070s with a cache of medical books in Arabic. He converted to Christianity, entered the Benedictine monastery of Monte Cassino, and spent the rest of his life translating his medical books into Latin. He translated about twenty texts, including works of Galen and the Hippocratic physicians as well as several Muslim physicians. One of the books Constantine translated was *Zād al-Musāfir* (*The Guide for the Traveler Going to Distant Countries*) by the Muslim physician Abū Ja'far Aḥmad ibn Ibrahim ibn Abi Khalid ibn al-Jazzār (d. 1009 CE), who practiced and taught medicine in the north African city of Al-Qayrawān in what is now Tunisia.[39] Constantine's Latin translation, titled the *Viaticum*, is a complete translation, with one significant omission. Constantine did not include the chapter "On Substances Which Induce Abortion and Kill the Seed in the Womb."[40] However, in translations of other Arabic medical texts, Constantine and his students did not omit material on contraception, even though contraception was also condemned by many theologians. Constantine's suppression of material on abortion was most likely due to theological objections to abortion. However, Monica Green points out that it is unique: "Even though it is quite likely that many extant early medieval medical manuscripts were written in monasteries or cathedral scriptoria, I have found no evidence for the suppression of discussions of abortifacients or other medical prescriptions that would equally conflict with orthodox Christian dogma."

his wife unconscious. When Dr. Wilcox arrived, Mrs. L was pale and clammy; her breathing was heavy, her pulse was "feeble and quick," and her extremities were cold. Her pupils did not contract when he shone light directly at them. Believing that she might have overdosed on opium, he forced an emetic down her throat every half hour and waited. After about three hours, Mrs. L began vomiting and regained consciousness. "The vomited matter," Wilcox observed, "consisted of liquid smelling strongly of pennyroyal."[46] When Mrs. L recovered enough to talk to the doctor, she told him she "had taken a teaspoonful of oil of pennyroyal" at nine in the evening before she went to bed. She had done this "in order to bring on her menses, which had been due several days." Dr. Wilcox made no comment on this, except to note that Mrs. L began menstruating on September 17. Pennyroyal is a species of mint with purple flowers. It smells like spearmint. And it has been used as an abortifacient for over two thousand years.

One interpretation of this story is that Mrs. L was trying to terminate a pregnancy. Because pennyroyal is toxic in large quantities, and because oil of pennyroyal is the most concentrated form one can ingest, Mrs. L's abortion nearly ended in her own death. Fortunately, her husband found her in time, and the doctor took quick action. The return of her menses indicates that, if she was pregnant before she swallowed the oil of pennyroyal and she wanted to not be pregnant, she succeeded, albeit with considerably more drama and discomfort than she might have hoped.

Dr. Wilcox never uses the word "abortion," and he had good reason not to. In 1825 Missouri had passed a law prohibiting the administration of drugs with intent to induce abortion.[47] Ten years later the law was amended to also prohibit the use of instruments to induce an abortion. The 1835 law drew a distinction between an abortion before quickening and after, making the former a lesser offence. The observation that Mrs. L's menstrual period was only "several days" late might be intended to signify that this abortion (if it was that) was well before quickening. If Mrs. L took oil of pennyroyal to terminate a pregnancy, she was part of a surge in the number of abortions in this period, and an increase in the number of married women seeking abortions. James Mohr summarizes this trend in his history of abortion in the United States:

> Before 1840 abortion was perceived in the United States primarily as a recourse of the desperate, especially of the young woman in trouble who feared the wrath of an over-exacting society. After 1840, however, evidence began to accumulate that the social character of the practice had changed. A high proportion of the women whose abortions contributed to the soaring incidence of that practice in the United States between 1840 and 1880 appeared to be married, native-born, Protestant women, frequently of middle- or upper-class status.[48]

This trend was deeply worrying to social conservatives who saw it as evidence of declining morals and a lack of proper maternal feeling among women. There was also a great deal of handwringing about the allegedly high fertility of immigrants and African Americans and the need for white, native-born Protestant women to save the nation from "race suicide" by devoting themselves to large families. In a Mother's Day speech in 1905, President Theodore Roosevelt opined that "if the average family in which there are children contained but two children the nation as a whole would decrease in population so rapidly that in two or three generations it would very deservedly be on the point of extinction, so that the people who had acted on this base and selfish doctrine would be giving place to others with braver and more robust ideals."[49] In other words, white women had a duty to the nation to procreate.

Lara Freidenfelds has demonstrated that, despite the constant exhortations from politicians, physicians, and preachers to breed like rabbits, many nineteenth-century American women were eager to limit their family sizes and to space out the births of their children. American women in the colonial and early Republican period had very high rates of fertility—an average of seven live births per woman—and valued large families. By contrast, married couples in the nineteenth century wanted fewer children and longer spaces between births. To achieve control over their fertility, they used a combination of contraceptives and "emmenagogues." They prolonged breastfeeding. And they resorted to abortion.[50] Mrs. L, already the mother of two young children, seems to fit this trend.

We do not know how Mrs. L procured oil of pennyroyal, but we do know that it would have been very easy to obtain. Pennyroyal, in various forms (pills, waters, wafers, teas, and oils) was sold at most pharmacists and via the mail. Most American newspapers in the nineteenth century carried advertisements for pennyroyal and other abortifacient substances, including rue and tansy, as well as for the services of abortionists.[51] Many of these substances, including pennyroyal, had a very long history of use as abortifacients. Ancient Greek and Roman medical texts include numerous drugs for inducing abortions, most of them made from plants, although animal parts were sometimes used as well.[52]

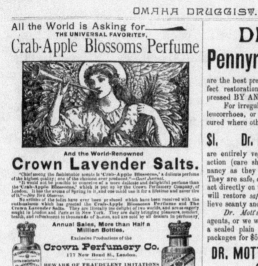
Ads published in *Omaha Druggist* 7, no. 4, April 1894. New York Academy of Medicine Library, New York, NY.

One Hippocratic technique to "bring down the menses" was to make a pessary of "pennyroyal, myrrh, frankincense, [and] bile of pig and bull" mixed with honey and insert it into the vagina.[53] The most famous of the Hippocratic texts, the oath, contains an explicit prohibition on doctors performing abortions. The oath reads, "I will not give an abortive pessary." The claim that Hippocrates forbade abortions at all stages of pregnancy for any reason still shows up on pro-life websites. But does the oath really ban all abortions? And how many physicians in the ancient world were bound by it? Helen King points out that the oath only prohibits a particular type of abortion, that induced using a pessary inserted into the vagina. This mode of delivery was more potent than taking an abortifacient drug orally. Per-

Many of the abortifacient herbs and plants described by Greek and Roman writers continued to show up in medical texts for the next two thousand years. The first English translation of Dioscorides's *De materia medica* was made by the botanist John Goodyer (1592–1664) and published in 1655. In his translation of Dioscorides's description of pennyroyal, Goodyer wrote that if a woman drinks pennyroyal tea it will "expelleth the menstrua, & the secunda [i.e., the placenta], & the Embrua."[64] Some early modern writers were cagier about the abortifacient properties of certain plants, especially in vernacular works that might reach a broader audience. In his *Complete Herbal*, also published in 1655, the physician Nicholas Culpeper (1616–1654) paraphrased Dioscorides's discussion of pennyroyal: "Being boiled and drank [pennyroyal] provokes women's courses and expels the dead child and afterbirth."[65] The botanist John Gerard (c. 1545–1612) made a similar alteration: "Pennie Royall boiled in wine and drunken, prouoketh the monthly termes, bringeth forth the secondine, the dead childe and vnnaturall birth."[66] Gerard also omits the abortifacient properties of rue: "The iuyce of Rue drunke with wine purgeth women after their deliuerance, driuing forth the secondine, the dead childe, and the vnnaturall birth."[67] Both men change Dioscorides's original "embryo" to "dead child," suggesting that pennyroyal and rue might be used to deal with an incomplete miscarriage or with a stillbirth. Nonetheless, it would not take a particularly astute reader to recognize that a drug that can expel a dead fetus can also expel a live one.

Historian John Riddle has pointed out that many of the plants used by the ancient Greeks and Romans to induce abortions really do contain chemicals that will terminate pregnancies. These plants include pennyroyal, rue, tansy, catnip, sage, myrtle, myrrh, and squirting cucumber. Pennyroyal and catnip, for

※ The time.

They flower about August, and somewhat later in colde sommers.

※ The names.

Masticke is called of the new writers *Marum* : of *Dioscorides Clinopodium. Dioscorides* sheweth that *Clinopodium* is οξύμελον, that is to say, a little shrub : of some it is called *Cleonicum*, and of the Latines *Lecispes*.

※ The nature.

These plants are hot and drie in the third degree.

※ The vertues.

Dioscorides writeth, that the herbe is drunke, and likewise the decoction thereof, against the bitings of venemous beasts, crampes and conuulsions, burstings and the strangurie. A

The decoction boiled in wine till the third part be consumed, and drunke, stoppeth the laske, in them that haue an ague, and vnto others in water. B

Of Pennie royall, or Pudding grasse.   Chap. 211.

1 *Pulegium regium.*
Pennie royall.

2 *Pulegium mas.*
Vpright Pennie royall.

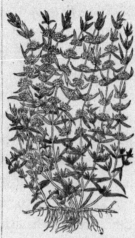
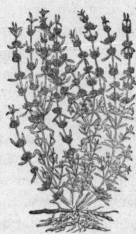

※ The description.

1 PVlegium regium vulgatum is so exceedingly well knowne to all our English nation, that it needeth no description, being our common Pennie roiall.

2   The second being the male Pennie roiall is like vnto the former, in leaues, flowers, and smell, and differeth in that this male kinde groweth vpright of himselfe without creeping, much like in shewe vnto wilde Marierome.

3   The thirde kinde of Pennie roiall groweth like vnto Time, and is of a wooddie substance, somewhat like vnto the thinne leafed Hyssope, of the fauour of common Pennie royall.

Mm I   3 *Pulegium*

example, both contain the organic compound pulegone, which is an abortifacient.[68] Riddle's work demonstrates that many premodern abortion drugs would produce the desired effect if taken in the correct amount. This is a big "if" though. The amount of pharmacologically active chemicals in plants varies according to season, soil, and other conditions. And some of these plants, like pennyroyal, can be toxic in large doses. While none of these drugs were foolproof and none were as effective as modern methods of contraception and abortion, they worked at least some of the time.

Since May 2022, when a draft of the *Dobbs v. Jackson Women's Health Organization* decision was leaked to the press and it became apparent that the US Supreme Court was about to overturn *Roe v. Wade*, there has been a surge of interest in the herbal abortifacients of the past. In June 2022, *Rolling Stone* magazine reported a dramatic increase in TikTok videos promoting herbal abortifacients. The article also noted that Google searches for pennyroyal, blue cohosh, and mugwort had "skyrocketed."[69] When I looked up the e-book version of *What to Expect When You're Expecting* on the Amazon website, I could view "popular highlights," which are passages that Kindle readers have highlighted. Over 1,200 Kindle readers have highlighted the following passage: "Pregnant women should particularly avoid the following oils, because some of them can trigger uterine contractions: basil, juniper, rosemary, sage, peppermint, pennyroyal, oregano, and thyme."[70]

In response, many physicians have pointed to the high toxicity of these substances and the very limited data on their efficacy. Pennyroyal, for example, can cause severe liver damage and death. Mrs. L's close call was no fluke; most people who ingest pennyroyal in a quantity sufficient to induce an abortion will end up vomiting and enduring abdominal pain if they do not slip into a coma and die. Mrs. L was lucky to survive, and her ordeal should make clear that herbal remedies are not necessarily "gentle" or "natural." The herbs used to induce abortion in the past were—and are—dangerous. Too high a dose and they were toxic; too low and they were ineffective.

The risks of abortifacient drugs were recognized in antiquity. The Hippocratic text *Epidemics* contains a graphic description of a woman who died in agony after taking an abortifacient drug:

> The wife of Simos had an abortion after 30 days. This happened either spontaneously, or after she drank something. Pain. Plenty of bilious, pale, green vomit every time she had something to drink. She had seizures, and she was biting her tongue. I visited on the fourth day, and her tongue was swollen and black. The white on her eyes was red. She was sleepless. On the fourth night she died.[71]

Historian Konstantinos Kapparis comments that both women and physicians in the ancient world recognized abortion as "perilously dangerous and painful."[72]

Many of the people dispensing information about herbal abortifacients make claims like, "Women have been using these herbs for centuries."[73] This is not entirely wrong. As we have seen, herbs like pennyroyal were described by the Hippocratic physicians. But the assumption that women in the past had some secret reserve of herbal lore that they used to manage their fertility before this knowledge was driven underground by modern medicine is categorically false. To be clear, some pre-modern women were skilled and respected healers, with extensive knowledge of the pharmacological properties of plants. And in many parts of the world, women turned to each other first for medical help in times of illness or crisis, especially in reproductive matters. But until the twentieth century, no medical practitioner, male or female, could provide truly safe and effective abortions. As we have seen, the notion that women know "secrets" about sex and reproduction, that they used and dispensed abortifacients under the noses of unsuspecting husbands and lovers, was a misogynistic projection of male fears, not a realistic description of reproductive health care in the past.

I stated that "one interpretation" of Dr. Wilcox's account of Mrs. L's case is that she took pennyroyal to terminate a pregnancy. I think, given the historical context, that this is most likely what was happening. But what should we make of her assertion that she was trying to "bring on her menses"? In the twenty-first century, this phrase sounds like a thinly veiled euphemism for inducing an abortion. Indeed, to us, the veil is so diaphanous as to be entirely transparent. But our views of menstruation are not the same as those of women in the nineteenth century, or earlier. We are more inclined to view a late period as a sign of pregnancy, whereas for earlier generations a missed period could mean many things. And we do not see a missed menstrual period as in and of itself a cause for concern.

If a woman today is trying to get pregnant and her period is late, she might begin to get excited. If she is trying not to get pregnant and has reason to believe her contraceptive method has failed, she might start to get worried. But if a woman is sure she is not pregnant and her period is late, she is unlikely to be overly concerned. She might attribute it to stress, unusual physical activity, jet lag, or the period goddess granting her a reprieve. What she is very *unlikely* to do is to take an emmenagogue, a medicine intended to provoke menstruation. But in the pre-modern world, regular menstruation was thought to be vital to a woman's health, and these views lingered on into the nineteenth century. It would have been entirely reasonable for a woman in the nineteenth century or earlier to be concerned that her menstrual period was late, even if she knew she was not pregnant. "Bringing on the menses" was still plausible enough in 1866 that Dr. Wilcox could publish the phrase in the *Boston Medical and Surgical Journal*, although his medical colleagues may well have read between the lines.

In pre-modern medicine, regular menstruation was seen as essential for a woman's general health but also for her fertility. Further, women were believed to be at their most fertile immediately after their menstrual periods. A woman might use a drug to induce menstruation to enhance her chances of getting pregnant. Or she might use it because she feared becoming seriously ill without the normal evacuation of menstrual blood from her body. Historian Etienne van de Walle suggests that the widespread acceptance of the importance of regular menstruation for women's health and fertility created a "zone of possibility" for women who wanted to end a pregnancy discreetly.[74] Brewing up a pot of tansy or pennyroyal tea would not necessarily signal to anyone that you were terminating a pregnancy.

Some historians have read "bring on the menses" as a euphemism for inducing an abortion. It is certainly true that many emmenagogues do contain plants now known to have abortifacient properties. For example, take a recipe to cure "retention of menses" from a medical book by the medieval nun Hildegard of Bingen:

Take rifelbere and about one-third as much yarrow, and aristologia, and about one-ninth as much rue, and crush this mixture in a mortar. Put it in a little bag and then cook it in wine; add clove and white pepper (a little less white pepper than clove) and honey. Drink this daily both fasting and with meals . . . for five days or fifteen, or until the matter is resolved.[75]

Aristologia, or aristolochia, is also known as birthwort. Dioscorides said birthwort could be made into a pessary that would bring down the menses or expel a dead fetus. Galen included it in a recipe for an abortifacient to be taken orally. Modern laboratory tests show that birthwort acts as both a contraceptive and an abortifacient.[76] And rue, as we have seen, is another known abortifacient. But was Hildegard really providing a coded recipe for ending a pregnancy? Most likely she was not.

Mrs. L's story draws us back into a world in which abortion care was intimately connected to other forms of health care for women. It shows us that the line between menstrual regulation and abortion was blurry, but we can push this insight further. Plants that were used to make abortifacient drugs almost always had multiple medical uses. They could also be used as contraceptives, as cures for infertility, and as "menstrual regulators," used to induce menstruation or to quell excessive menstrual bleeding. For example, the ancient Greeks used pennyroyal as an abortifacient, but also a contraceptive, a fertility aid, and a menstrual regulator. Aristophanes's plays *Peace* and *Lysistrata* both allude to the contraceptive uses of pennyroyal, suggesting that his audience would have been familiar with them.[77] One Hippocratic text says that a woman can increase her chances of getting pregnant if she drinks "pennyroyal in juniper-wine" before having sex with her husband.[78] It might seem peculiar to use the same herb as a contraceptive, a cure for infertility, and discussed separately, as though restriction of abortion has no implications for other reproductive health services (it does). Abortion care is usually delivered in separate places. Most hospitals do not offer abortion services; most obstetricians and gynecologists do not perform abortions. Abortion has become a highly specialized medical service. This blinds us to the fact that there is considerable overlap between abortion care and other reproductive health services. If a woman goes to a hospital because she is miscarrying, the treatment she will be given to ensure that the miscarriage goes to completion is in many cases the same drugs and procedures that would be used to perform an abortion.[83] The overlap between abortion and miscarriage management has had dire consequences in Catholic health care facilities. Catholic hospitals in the US and elsewhere have consistently refused to perform abortions, even when the fetus is nonviable and even when the life of the mother is at risk.[84]

One of the most dramatic and well-publicized examples of this kind of policy is the case of Savita Halappanavar in Ireland. Halappanavar died in a Galway hospital of a septic miscarriage in October 2012. Her death was clearly preventable. She entered the hospital because she was having a miscarriage at seventeen weeks. She was told that it was impossible to save the fetus, at which point she requested a therapeutic abortion. Doctors refused because there was a detectable fetal heartbeat. They withheld medical treatment for several days until Halappanavar finally miscarried on her own. By this point she had developed sepsis and her condition had deteriorated so far that it was impossible to save her life.[85] Halappanavar's tragic death made brutally clear what happens when the life of the fetus is so infinitely precious that extending this life as long as possible, even if only a few days, is worth any price, up to and including the mother's life. And it highlights what can go wrong when abortion care and miscarriage care are treated as two radically distinct medical services.

Cases like Halappanavar's have multiplied in the United States since *Roe* was overturned.[86] In states with abortion bans, doctors and hospital administrators are now making women with ectopic pregnancies—which are always nonviable and always life-threatening for the pregnant person—wait until their treatment is approved by hospital boards and lawyers, creating potentially deadly delays. Doctors and hospital administrators are also refusing to treat women who are miscarrying if their fetuses still have a heartbeat. This is precisely the scenario that led to Halappanavar's death from sepsis. Although most abortion bans have exceptions for "medical emergencies," when the pregnant person's life is at risk, just what constitutes an acceptable level of risk is unclear. Physicians and hospital administrators are currently reluctant to intervene unless the risk is very high, for fear of prosecution if their judgment is challenged. It is only a matter of time before deaths like Halappanavar's become common in the United States.

CONCLUSION

In the late twentieth and early twenty-first centuries, many women have spoken or written publicly about their abortions, and several organizations actively solicit and collect such stories.[87] For the recent past, we finally have a rich and growing trove of sources about abortion from the "uterus-carrying perspective." The multitude of modern stories, each one different because each pregnant person's life is different, stands in stark contrast to the paucity of sources for the more distant past. While we cannot recover the voices and experiences of people in the past who had abortions, willingly or not, we can at least acknowledge that those voices and experiences were as varied as those of the present. Pro-life arguments still invoke the age-old stereotype of women who seek abortions as irresponsible sluts. They do this because male writers since antiquity have flattened all abortion-seeking women into projections of their own anxieties. When we look at stories of abortion in the past, like the stories of the slave, the princess, and the mother that I highlighted in this chapter, we should recognize that there was always more to these women's lives than male authors imagined.

CONCLUSION

began writing this book when Donald Trump was president. It was clear from the day of his surprise victory over Hillary Clinton that reproductive rights were in danger. A substantial portion of Trump's base were (and are) evangelical Christians who expected him to abolish legal abortion. During his presidency, pro-life politicians and activists were emboldened to push for more restrictive abortion laws in many states. These included "heartbeat laws" that ban abortion after a fetal "heartbeat" is detected and "fetal personhood laws" that define a fertilized egg as a human being. These laws do not just ban abortion, they also justify the regulation of pregnant people and the criminalization of actions perceived as detrimental to the fetus. As Alison McCulloch writes, "Once you have a citizen, a person, living inside you, with all the rights and moral status that citizenship and personhood attract, then the authorities gain the right of entry, and a regulatory role in how that fetal citizen is treated."[1] In the interests of "protecting" the fetus, the mother's rights to privacy and bodily autonomy can be abrogated. Trump's appointment of two Catholic pro-life judges to the US Supreme Court put the final nails in the coffin of *Roe v. Wade*.

Like many Americans, I could see that I was witnessing a period of rapid historical change as the rights that I enjoyed throughout my reproductive years were stripped away from my children's generation. But as a historian who has spent the past three decades studying and teaching the history of reproduction, I could also see that I was witnessing arguments and ideas that were very old indeed. Although heartbeat laws and fetal personhood laws are specific to the twentieth and twenty-first centuries, I often experienced a sense of déjà vu when I read or heard support for these bills.

One of those moments of déjà vu came when I read an exchange on Twitter between Congresswoman Alexandria Ocasio-Cortez of New York and conservative commentator Liz Wheeler. Although this exchange occurred in response to the passage of a heartbeat bill, it fits seamlessly into the long history of separating accounts of fetal development from accounts of pregnancy. On May 7, 2019, after Georgia governor Brian Kemp signed a bill banning abortion after a fetal heartbeat can be detected, that is, at about six weeks, Ocasio-Cortez tweeted: "'6 weeks pregnant'=2 weeks late on your period. Most of the men writing these bills don't know the first thing about a woman's body outside of the things they want from it. It's relatively common for a woman to have a late period + not be pregnant."[2] Wheeler responded to the tweet with a picture of an embryo and the comment: "This is 'two weeks late on your period.' Two weeks late has arms & legs forming, fingers & toes, & a heartbeat!"[3]

In her response to the Georgia legislation, Ocasio-Cortez centered women's experiences. A late period could mean pregnancy, but it could also mean stress or illness or change in diet or a thousand other things or nothing at all. And "late," when talking about menstruation, is relative. A woman with very regular periods might notice when it is a day or two late; a woman with irregular periods might not notice the absence of her period for several weeks. Six weeks is still in the murky realm of the late period and ambiguous home pregnancy test results. Six weeks is well before most obstetricians will even see patients, let alone monitor them. And a high percentage of early pregnancies end in miscarriage. At six weeks a woman's uterus is like Schrödinger's famous thought experiment with the cat in the box—where the possibilities are missed period, miscarriage, and viable pregnancy.[4] Many women do not know they are pregnant until well after this point.

Wheeler centered the fetus. Her tweet assumes that a missed period can only mean pregnancy and that pregnancy should be described solely in terms of embryonic and fetal development. During the sixth week of pregnancy, the embryo is beginning to develop features that we recognize as human. Her choice to highlight arms and fingers is not accidental, as these terms are used almost exclusively to describe human appendages. Animals may have legs, toes, and hearts, but only humans have opposable thumbs. Why, I wondered when I read Wheeler's tweet, are we still linking the personhood of the fetus to its humanlike appearance? Why does the image she posted to accompany the tweet look so much like the fetuses in bottles collected by Frederik Ruysch in the seventeenth century?

The separation between pregnancy and fetal development, and the persistent fear that the interests of the pregnant woman and the fetus are in conflict, has deep roots in the histories of medicine, science, religion, and philosophy. Placing debates about reproduction in historical context helps us to understand why our laws and policies have such profoundly negative consequences for the health of mothers and babies.

I finished this book a few months after the *Dobbs v. Jackson Women's Health Organization* decision. Although the full consequences have yet to unfold, its effects will extend into all areas of health care for women, trans men, and nonbinary people who were assigned female at birth. Already, doctors and pharmacists have started denying women with lupus and rheumatoid arthritis methotrexate, the drug that is the "gold standard" for managing these conditions. Methotrexate is also used to end ectopic pregnancies. Should a person become pregnant while on the drug, it would likely cause an abortion.[5] Neurologists have raised concerns about how new restrictions on abortion will impact the treatment of women with migraines, multiple sclerosis (MS), and epilepsy, because the drugs used can have teratogenic effects. "In a climate of increased limitations on reproductive rights, whereby pregnancies cannot be reliably timed or prevented," writes Dr. Sara LaHue, "neurologists might possibly restrict use of the effective medications that are standard care for other patient groups because of potential concerns about causing fetal harm."[6] Oncologists, too, have pointed out that the options for treating pregnant people with cancer may be severely compromised by laws intended to protect fetuses.[7] All of these examples indicate that, in many states, the protection of "potential life" will mean the privileging of potential life over actual life.

While I have traced continuities in thinking about reproduction from the ancient world to the present, I do not mean to suggest that because some of our ideas are very old that they are natural or inevitable. My point is precisely the opposite. Uncovering the histories of these ideas—about fetal heartbeats, about men playing the active role in the creation of offspring, about the dangers of the uterine environment, and about the malicious tendency of some women to secretly abort their fetuses—is a first step to understanding that they are neither natural nor inevitable. We could find ways of thinking about pregnant people and fetuses that respect the dignity, and foster the well-being, of both.

I noted at the beginning of this book that it was not a comprehensive history of embryology. I chose to focus on aspects of that history that were relevant to contemporary issues, but also ones that display the continuities between the past and the present. Another value to studying history is that we encounter ways of thinking that are different from our own. Examining unfamiliar ideas about procreation can cast new light on our own assumptions. For example, based on her analysis of seventeenth-century English medical texts, historian Mary Fissell found that many English people in this period imagined the fetus "as a sort of guest within the mother's body, and it was her job to provide appropriate hospitality to it, just as she would in her own home." In this metaphor, "women's bodies were naturally welcoming and generous."[8] This way of thinking about pregnancy is, as she points out, strange to modern readers. We are far more accustomed to metaphors that imply that pregnant women's bodies are passive. And, as I have demonstrated in this book, we have deeply ingrained fears of the dangers posed to the fetus by the pregnant woman.

The implication of saying a woman has a "guest in her house" is very different than saying she has a "bun in the oven." Taking care of a guest is work, but it is work that one undertakes willingly and (ideally) lovingly. If you are forced to take someone into your house and care for them, they are not a guest. Hospitality is also embedded in notions of community, reciprocity, and mutual obligations. By contrast, the metaphor of the bun in the oven implies that the womb is nothing more than a heat source. The real work of creating the fetus has already been done by the father. The point is not that one metaphor is more "accurate" than the other—both capture some aspects of pregnancy and ignore others. The point is that the "guest in the house" metaphor forms the basis for a more positive view of pregnancy, and of the pregnant woman, than does the "bun in the oven" metaphor. If we thought of women's bodies as inherently nurturing, rather than inherently dangerous, we would be less likely to blame and to punish women for poor pregnancy outcomes. If we thought of pregnancy as creative work, rather than incubation, we would be more likely to support and nurture pregnant people.

ACKNOWLEDGMENTS

Having examined two thousand years of metaphors for pregnancy and fetal development, I hope the reader will indulge me as I reflect on the "gestation" of the book and offer my gratitude to the people who sustained me during the writing process. This book is a product of the happy marriage of my research and teaching. I first became interested in the history of reproduction in graduate school under the guidance of Mary Fissell, who has served as a mentor, role model, and friend for almost three decades. Every page bears the imprint of her scholarship, advice, and encouragement. I have presented material from the manuscript at academic conferences and workshops at the Herzog August Library in Wolfenbüttel, Germany, and the Huntington Library in San Marino, California, and at meetings of Scientiae and the American Association for the History of Medicine. I am grateful to the audiences and participants at these events who provided suggestions, references, and avenues of inquiry that have immeasurably improved the finished work.

I have been teaching history of medicine at the University of Oklahoma for the past twenty years, talking to undergraduates in one of the reddest states in the country about the history of pregnancy, childbirth, contraception, and abortion. Over the years, I have used a great deal of the material in this book in my classes, and I owe an enormous debt to my students. I do not think I would have written this book if I had not read so many course evaluations with variations of "I expected to find the pre-modern history boring, but it was actually fascinating." My students pushed me to explain strange concepts more clearly and to articulate how learning about the past could help us forge a better present and future. And they energized me with their curiosity, idealism, generosity, tenacity, and passion.

I have written two short essays on material from this book for *Nursing Clio*, a blog created by Jacqueline Antonovich that provides a public forum for historical scholarship on contemporary issues in medicine and gender. I am indebted to the editors who worked with me on these pieces and helped me to refine my ideas, especially Laura Ansley and R. E. Fulton. Beyond this, I am grateful to all the *Nursing Clio* editors and contributors for creating a vibrant public conversation about the historical roots of contemporary debates on women's bodies and women's health care. Their work has been a model for this book.

I could not have had a better editor than Matt McAdam of Johns Hopkins University Press. His advice on both content and style have made this a much better, and more readable, book than I could have produced otherwise. Three anonymous reviewers for Hopkins Press offered incisive criticism tempered with enthusiastic encouragement, and I am grateful for both.

Bridging the personal and professional, my husband, Peter Barker, read and commented on drafts of chapters and has supported me in a thousand ways, big and small, through the writing process. Our four children, Karen, Erika, Max, and Niels, are a constant source of joy and inspiration. It is to them that this book is lovingly dedicated.

FURTHER READING

For readers interested in delving deeper into some of the topics in this book, there is a wealth of material. The following recommendations are aimed at general readers and include, for the most part, books and articles that are in English and accessible to nonspecialists.

HISTORY OF REPRODUCTION

The most comprehensive work on the history of reproduction is *Reproduction: Antiquity to the Present Day*, a collection of essays edited by Nick Hopwood, Rebecca Flemming, and Lauren Kassell (Cambridge: Cambridge University Press, 2018). The contributors to this volume are experts in a wide range of topics, periods, and geographical areas. The book covers gestation and childbirth, fertility and infertility, abortion and contraception, eugenics and population control, and more, moving from the Ancient Near East to the twenty-first century.

There are also many wonderful studies of reproduction in particular times and places. For ancient Greek ideas about procreation and women's bodies, see Helen King, *Hippocrates' Woman: Reading the Female Body in Ancient Greece* (London: Routledge, 1998). On re-production in the Middle Ages, see Joan Cadden, *Meanings of Sex Difference in the Middle Ages* (Cambridge: Cambridge University Press, 1993), and Monica H. Green, *Making Women's Medicine Masculine: The Rise of Male Authority in Pre-Modern Gynaecology* (Oxford: Oxford University Press, 2008). For the early modern period, see Barbara Duden, *The Woman Beneath the Skin: A Doctor's Patients in Eighteenth-Century Germany*, translated by Thomas Dunlap (Cambridge, MA: Harvard University Press, 1991); Mary E. Fissell, *Vernacular Bodies: The Politics of Reproduction in Early Modern England* (Oxford: Oxford University Press, 2007); and Cathy McClive, *Menstruation and Procreation in Early Modern France* (Burlington, VT: Ashgate, 2015).

Histories of reproduction in modern America are more numerous. Out of a rich bounty, I have selected four books, each of which explores different aspects of reproductive medicine and politics in the United States. Judith Walzer Leavitt's *Brought to Bed: Childbearing in America, 1750 to 1950* (Oxford: Oxford University Press, 1986) examines the medical and social practices surrounding childbirth between the mid-eighteenth and the mid-twentieth centuries, covering the shift from home births involving midwives to hospital births involving physicians.

Sara Dubow's *Ourselves Unborn: A History of the Fetus in Modern America* (Oxford: Oxford University Press, 2011) charts changing ideas about the fetus between the late nineteenth and the early twenty-first centuries, including the rise of the concept of fetal personhood. Rickie Solinger's *Pregnancy and Power: A Short History of Reproductive Politics in America* (New York: New York University Press, 2005) examines laws, policies, and social attitudes toward reproduction and the control of reproduction from the late eighteenth century to the end of the twentieth century, paying particular attention to the ways race and class shaped the reproductive experiences of American girls and women. Finally, Dorothy Roberts's groundbreaking *Killing the Black Body: Race, Reproduction, and the Meaning of Liberty*, 2nd ed. (New York: Penguin Random House, 2017) centers Black women's experiences, examining the myriad ways in which Black women in America have been denied reproductive autonomy and dignity, from the sexual exploitation and forced pregnancies of enslaved women, to coercive sterilizations, to the moral panic surrounding crack babies and welfare queens.

DISSECTING AND COLLECTING FETAL SPECIMENS

Katharine Park's foundational work on the origins of anatomical dissection in Europe, *Secrets of Women: Gender, Generation, and the Origins of Human Dissection* (New York: Zone Books, 2006), demonstrates the intense interest in cutting open the female body, especially the uterus, during the late Middle Ages. Desire to see the mysteries of human procreation spurred the dissections of female cadavers as well as fetuses and neonates. There is, unfortunately, no book on Frederik Ruysch or any other anatomist who collected and preserved fetal specimens in the seventeenth and eighteenth centuries. But there are two fascinating articles on Ruysch and his preparations: Rina Knoeff, "Touching Anatomy: On the Handling of Preparations in the Anatomical Cabinets of Frederik Ruysch (1638–1731)," *Studies in History and Philosophy of Science Part C: Studies in History and Philosophy of Biological and Biomedical Sciences* 49 (2015): 32–44, and Dániel Margócsy, "Advertising Cadavers in the Republic of Letters: Anatomical Publications in the Early Modern Netherlands," *British Journal for the History of Science* 42, no. 2 (2009): 187–210. In *Icons of Life: A Cultural History of Human Embryos* (Berkeley: University of California Press, 2009), Lynn Morgan traces the career and collecting practices of Franklin Mall, professor of anatomy at the Johns Hopkins University Medical School, who established the largest embryo collection in the United States. Mall's collection formed the basis of the Carnegie Human Embryo Collection, which is still used by embryologists.

MISCARRIAGE

There are two excellent recent histories of miscarriage in America: Shannon Withycombe, *Lost: Miscarriage in Nineteenth-Century America* (New Brunswick, NJ: Rutgers University Press, 2018), and Lara Freidenfelds, *The Myth of the Perfect Pregnancy: A History of Miscarriage in America* (New York: Oxford University Press, 2020). Both demonstrate that attitudes toward miscarriage have changed dramatically over the last hundred years and that in the past, American women did not generally perceive a miscarriage as the loss of a child. There has been less work on miscarriage in earlier periods, but Barbara Duden touches on the subject in *The Woman Beneath the Skin: A Doctor's Patients in Eighteenth-Century Germany*, translated by Thomas Dunlap (Cambridge, MA: Harvard University Press, 1991).

MATERNAL-FETAL CONFLICT

The concept of maternal-fetal conflict has been studied extensively. Important books on the subject include Elizabeth M. Armstrong, *Conceiving Risk, Bearing Responsibility: Fetal Alcohol Syndrome and the Diagnosis of Moral Disorder* (Baltimore: Johns Hopkins University Press, 2003); Jeanne Flavin, *Our Bodies, Our Crimes: The Policing of Women's Reproduction in America* (New York: New York University Press, 2009); and Sheena Meredith, *Policing Pregnancy: The Law and Ethics of Obstetric Conflict* (Burlington, VT: Ashgate, 2005).

On the criminalization of miscarriage, see Michelle Goldberg, "When a Miscarriage Is Manslaughter," *New York Times*, October 18, 2021, https://www.nytimes.com/2021/10/18/opinion/poolaw -miscarriage.html, and New York Times Editorial Board, "When Prosecutors Jail a Mother for a Miscarriage," *New York Times*,

December 28, 2018, https://www.nytimes.com/interactive/2018/12 /28/opinion/abortion-pregnancy-pro-life.html.

On the hysteria surrounding drug use in pregnant women, see Nina Martin, "Take a Valium, Lose Your Kid, Go to Jail," ProPublica, September 23, 2015, https://www.propublica.org/article/when-the -womb-is-a-crime-scene, and New York Times Editorial Board, "Slandering the Unborn," *New York Times*, December 28, 2018, https://www.nytimes.com/interactive/2018/12/28/opinion/crack -babies-racism.html.

MATERNAL MORBIDITY AND MORTALITY

The unusually high rates of maternal morbidity and mortality in the United States have attracted considerable attention in the last few years. Recent analyses of the problem include Commonwealth Fund, "Policies for Reducing Maternal Morbidity and Mortality and Enhancing Equity in Maternal Health: A Review of the Evidence," November 16, 2021, https://www.commonwealthfund.org /publications/fund-reports/2021/nov/policies-reducing-maternal -morbidity-mortality-enhancing-equity#6, and Nina Martin and Renee Montagne, "The Last Person You'd Expect to Die in Childbirth," ProPublica and NPR, May 12, 2017, https://www.propublica.org /article/die-in-childbirth-maternal-death-rate-health-care-system.

Black women are more than twice as likely to die from pregnancy-related conditions. For the historic roots of the racial disparity in maternal mortality and morbidity rates, see Dorothy Roberts, *Killing the Black Body: Race, Reproduction, and the Meaning of Liberty*, 2nd ed. (New York: Penguin Random House, 2017). For analyses of Black maternal mortality in the twenty-first century, see Nina Martin and Renee Montagne, "Nothing Protects Black Women from Dying in Pregnancy and Childbirth," ProPublica and NPR, December 7, 2017, https://www.propublica.org/article/nothing-protects -black-women-from-dying-in-pregnancy-and-childbirth, and Myra J. Tucker, Cynthia J. Berg, William M. Callaghan, and Jason Hsia, "The

Black-White Disparity in Pregnancy-Related Mortality from 5 Conditions: Differences in Prevalence and Case-Fatality Rates," *American Journal of Public Health* 97, no. 2 (2007): 247–251. Monica J. Casper's *Babylost: Racism, Survival, and the Quiet Politics of Infant Mortality, from A to Z* (New Brunswick, NJ: Rutgers University Press, 2022) focuses on the disproportionately high rates of mortality among Black infants, but much of her analysis is directly relevant to racial differences in maternal mortality and morbidity.

ABORTION

Multiple historians have written histories of abortion in the United States, analyzing the legal, political, religious, and social aspects. The four that I have found most useful are Jennifer L. Holland, *Tiny You: A Western History of the Anti-Abortion Movement* (Oakland: University of California Press, 2020); James C. Mohr, *Abortion in America: The Origins and Evolution of National Policy, 1800–1900* (New York: Oxford University Press, 1978); Leslie J. Reagan, *When Abortion Was a Crime: Women, Medicine, and Law in the United States, 1867–1973* (Berkeley: University of California Press, 1997); and Rickie Solinger, ed., *Abortion Wars: A Half Century of Struggle, 1950–2000* (Berkeley: University of California Press, 1998).

In addition, there are several works on abortion in earlier periods. On the legal, medical, and moral dimensions of abortion in ancient Greece and Rome, see Konstantinos Kapparis, *Abortion in the Ancient World* (London: Duckworth, 2002). On methods of inducing abortion in antiquity, see John M. Riddle, *Eve's Herbs: A History of Contraception and Abortion in the West* (Cambridge, MA: Harvard University Press, 1997). Tara Mulder has written a couple of short, thoughtful pieces on ancient attitudes toward abortion and fetal personhood and their relevance to contemporary debates about abortion: "The Hippocratic Oath in *Roe v. Wade*," *Eidolon*, March 10, 2016, https://eidolon.pub/the-hippocratic-oath-in-roe-v-wade-ded59eedfd8f, and "Ancient Medicine and Fetal Per-

sonhood," *Eidolon,* October 26, 2015, https://eidolon.pub/ancient
-medicine-and-the-straw-man-of-fetal-personhood-73eed36b945a#
.3n2a1fqm3.

Medieval historians have shown that, contrary to popular belief, Christians were not universally opposed to abortion. See Zu-
bin Mistry, *Abortion in the Early Middle Ages c. 500–900* (Suffolk: York
Medieval Press, 2015); Maeve Callan, "Saints Once Did Abortions—It
Was a Lesser Sin than Oral Sex," *Irish Times,* April 19, 2018, https://
www.irishtimes.com/culture/books/saints-once-did-abortions-it
-was-a-lesser-sin-than-oral-sex-1.3466881, and Luis Josué Salés, "As
Texas Ban on Abortion Goes into Effect, a Religion Scholar Explains
That Pre-Modern Christian Attitudes on Marriage and Reproductive
Rights Were Quite Different," *The Conversation,* September 2, 2021,
https://theconversation.com/as-texas-ban-on-abortion-goes-into
-effect-a-religion-scholar-explains-that-pre-modern-christian-atti
tudes-on-marriage-and-reproductive-rights-were-quite-different
-167170.

NOTES

INTRODUCTION

1. *Roe v. Wade.*
2. *Dobbs v. Jackson Women's Health Organization.*
3. Guttmacher Institute, "State Bans on Abortion throughout Pregnancy."
4. Taylor, *The Public Life of the Fetal Sonogram*; Valvoline commercial (2000), https://www.youtube.com/watch?v=GfUzQZOVufo; Doritos commercial, Super Bowl 50 (2016), https://www.postcrescent.com /story/entertainment/television/2016/02/08/watch-super-bowl-50-ads /80002876/.
5. Casper, *The Making of the Unborn Patient.*
6. Armstrong, *Conceiving Risk, Bearing Responsibility.*
7. Oaks, "Smoke-Filled Wombs and Fragile Fetuses," 63–108.
8. Paltrow and Flavin, "Arrests of and Forced Interventions on Pregnant Women," 299–343.
9. Meredith, *Policing Pregnancy*; Morris, *Cut It Out*, esp. chap. 5.
10. New York Times Editorial Board, "When Prosecutors Jail a Mother for a Miscarriage"; Aspinwall, Bailey, and Yurkanin, "They Lost Pregnancies for Unclear Reasons."

1   THE TELL-TALE HEART

1. Najmabadi, "Fetal 'Heartbeat' Bill." For the text of Texas Senate Bill 8, see https://legiscan.com/TX/text/SB8/2021.

2. Slawson, "Heartbeat Act—Open (SS)." Slawson posted a video of her speech on her Facebook page on May 19, 2021. All quotes from the speech are my own transcription of this video.

3. Jauhar, *Heart*, 23.

4. It is no longer on the front page of the website, but Porter has made this statement before. See for example Porter, "Should Ohio Prohibit Abortions after Six Weeks?"

5. Faith2Action, "The Pro-Life Heartbeat Bill."

6. Eckholm, "Anti-Abortion Groups Are Split on Legal Tactics."

7. Quoted in Eckholm, "Anti-Abortion Groups Are Split on Legal Tactics."

8. Evans and Narasimhan, "A Narrative Analysis of Anti-Abortion Testimony," 215.

9. Szoch, *The Best Pro-Life Arguments for Secular Audiences*.

10. Szoch, *The Best Pro-Life Arguments for Secular Audiences*, 1.

11. Szoch, *The Best Pro-Life Arguments for Secular Audiences*, 5.

12. Glenza, "Doctors' Organization: Calling Abortion Bans 'Fetal Heartbeat Bills' Is Misleading." In medical terms, the beginning of a pregnancy is the first day of the pregnant person's last menstrual period.

13. Simmons-Duffin, "The Texas Abortion Ban Hinges On 'Fetal Heartbeat.'"

14. Both quoted in Najmabadi, "Fetal 'Heartbeat' Bill."

15. This is true of Texas S.B. 8 and Oklahoma H.B. 2441. For the text of Texas Senate Bill 8, see https://legiscan.com/TX/text/SB8/2021; for the text of Oklahoma House Bill 2441, see http://oklegislature.gov/BillInfo .aspx?Bill=HB2441.

16. Aristotle, *On the Soul*. See also Park, "The Organic Soul," 464–484.

17. Aristotle, *On the Parts of Animals*.

18. Hurlbutt, "*Peri Kardies*," 1112.

19. Aristotle, *On the Parts of Animals*.

20. *Harry Potter and the Chamber of Secrets*. This line is in the film but not the book.

21. Aristotle, *On the Parts of Animals*.

22. Aristotle, *On the Parts of Animals*.

23. Hankinson, "Galen's Anatomy of the Soul," 198.

24. Flemming, "Galen's Generations of Seeds," 95–108.

25. Galen, *On the Doctrines of Hippocrates and Plato*, quoted in Hankinson, "Galen's Anatomy of the Soul," p. 200, n. 12.

26. Hankinson, "Galen's Anatomy of the Soul," 208.

27. Flemming, "Galen's Generations of Seeds," 102–103.

28. Berger, *Hildegard of Bingen*, 74.
29. Webb, *Medieval Heart*, 42.
30. Albert the Great, *De animalibus*, quoted in Webb, *Medieval Heart*, 26.
31. Webb, *Medieval Heart*, 97.
32. Demaitre, *Medieval Medicine*, 233.
33. "Cor irascibilis, seu vindictae honorisque concupiscibilis animae se- dem esse, Hippocrati, Platoni, Galeno, & Stoicis ac Peripateticis pariter omnibus concessum fuit." Vesalius, *De humani corporis fabrica*, 594.
34. "spiritus vitalis fontem, & caloris nativi sedem fomitemque." Vesa- lius, *De humani corporis fabrica*, 595.
35. "vitalis caloris fons." Colombo, *De re anatomica*, 175.
36. Harvey, *The Circulation of the Blood*, 3.
37. "The Case of a Man," 347.
38. "The Case of a Man," 353.
39. Donald Effler, "Surgery for Coronary Disease," *Scientific American* 210 (October 1968): 43. Quoted in Jones, *Broken Hearts*, 8.
40. Marmot et al., "Health Inequalities among British Civil Servants," 1387–1393.
41. Greenwood, Carnahan, and Huang, "Patient-physician gender con- cordance," 8569–8574.
42. Boyle, "Broken Hearts," 731–732.
43. Matthew 5:8 and 15:19 (King James Version).
44. Boyle, "Broken Hearts."
45. Saint Augustine, *The Confessions of Saint Augustine*.
46. Park, *Secrets of Women*, 41.
47. Bouley, *Pious Postmortems*, 62.
48. Bouley, *Pious Postmortems*, 116.
49. Karant-Nunn, "Martin Luther's Heart," in *The Personal Luther*, 158, 160.
50. Quoted in Karant-Nunn "Martin Luther's Heart," 163.
51. Calvin, *Institutes of the Christian Religion*, 30.
52. *The Book of Common Prayer—1549*.
53. King, "A Tough Mind and a Tender Heart."
54. Graham, *Hope for the Troubled Heart*.
55. Spadaro, "A Big Heart Open to God."
56. Curry, "Bishop Michael Curry's Royal Wedding Sermon."
57. Slawson, "Heartbeat Act—Open (SS)."
58. Edgar, "The Rhetoric of Auscultation," 351–352.
59. Marshall, "Ultrasound Images of Two Fetuses Shown to Lawmakers." See also Edgar, "The Rhetoric of Auscultation," 350.

60. Marshall, "Fetuses to Be Presented as Witnesses."
61. Dickson, "Fetus to Testify against Abortion."
62. Carmon, "Fetus To 'Testify' in Support of Ohio Heartbeat Bill."
63. Carmon, "Ohio Fetus Testimony Doesn't Go So Well."
64. Wolf, *Cesarean Section*.
65. Wolf, *Cesarean Section*, 127 and 166.
66. Wolf, *Cesarean Section*, 149.
67. Wolf, *Cesarean Section*, 165.
68. Wolf, *Cesarean Section*, 165.
69. Wolf, *Cesarean Section*, 165–166.
70. Wolf, *Cesarean Section*, 165.
71. Wolf, *Cesarean Section*, 166.
72. The story was originally published in *Pioneer* magazine in January 1843.
73. Dickson, "Fetus to Testify against Abortion."

2   THE FETUS IN THE BOTTLE

1. Cleveland Clinic, "Am I Pregnant?"
2. Buzzfeed, "23 Extremely Difficult Side Effects of Pregnancy."
3. Healthline, "Weird Early Pregnancy Symptoms No One Tells You About."
4. CNET, "10 Weird Pregnancy Symptoms That Are Totally Normal."
5. Lucy Huber (@clhubes), Twitter, September 3, 2022, https://twitter.com/clhubes/status/1566062420635930624.
6. Bates, *Everyday Sexism*, 266–267.
7. Szoch, *The Best Pro-Life Arguments for Secular Audiences*, 5.
8. Holland, *Tiny You*, 55.
9. Kapparis, *Abortion in the Ancient World*, 33–52, quote on p. 36.
10. Aristotle, *History of Animals*, 437.
11. von Staden, "The Discovery of the Body," 223–241; Gleason, "Shock and Awe," 85–114.
12. Hippocrates, *Eight Months Child*, quoted in Hanson, "The Eight Months' Child," 594.
13. Aristotle, *History of Animals*; Aristotle, *Parts of Animals*; Aristotle, *Generation of Animals*.
14. Aristotle, *On the Soul*. See also Park, "The Organic Soul," 464–484.
15. Aristotle, *Generation of Animals*, 109.
16. Aristotle, *Generation of Animals*, 11.
17. Aristotle, *Generation of Animals*, 121.

18. Aristotle, *Generation of Animals*, 133.

19. Cheung, "Madison Cawthorn, Accused Sexual Harasser"; Boboltz, "Madison Cawthorn Thinks Your Pregnancy Is A Polaroid."

20. *Generation* and *Nature of the Child* in Hippocrates, *Generation. Nature of the Child. Diseases 4. Nature of Women and Barrenness*, 1–23 and 25–93.

21. Hippocrates, *Generation*, 15–17.

22. Hippocrates, *Nature of the Child*, 31–35.

23. Hippocrates, *Nature of the Child*, 45.

24. Hippocrates, *Nature of the Child*, 51.

25. Hanson, "The Eight Months' Child," 596.

26. Flemming, "Galen's Generations of Seeds," 95

27. Über die Ausformung der Keimlinge zu schreiben, haben sowohl Ärzte als auch Philosophen unternommen, ohne daß sie für ihre Aussagen irgendeinen Anhaltspunkt aus der Anatomie bieten. Galen, *Galeni De foetuum formatione*, 55.

28. Hankinson, "Galen's Anatomy of the Soul," 198.

29. Galen, *On the Doctrines of Hippocrates and Plato*, quoted in Hankinson, "Galen's Anatomy of the Soul," 200, n. 12.

30. Hankinson, "Galen's Anatomy of the Soul," 208.

31. Flemming, "Galen's Generations of Seeds," 102–103.

32. Noor, "What a Pregnancy Actually Looks Like."

33. MYA Network, "The Issue of Tissue."

34. Snyder, "Guardian Article 'What a Pregnancy Actually Looks Like' Erases Embryos."

35. Heipel, "The *Guardian* Is Wrong."

36. On medieval embryology, see Cadden, *Meanings of Sex Difference*, esp. pp. 88–104; Lemay, *Women's Secrets*, esp. pp. 63–95; and Dunstan, *The Human Embryo*.

37. Park, *Secrets of Women*, 81.

38. The incident is described in Ladurie, *The Beggar and the Professor*, chap. 6.

39. Jimenez, "The First Autopsy in the New World," 618–619.

40. Platter, *De corporis humani structura et usu*, tabula 3.

41. Bauhin, *Theatrum anatomicum*.

42. Zerbi, *Opus preclarum anathomie totius corporis humani*. For biographical information on Zerbi, see Lind, *Studies in Pre-Vesalian Anatomy*, 1–18.

43. "De generatione embrionis," in Zerbi, *Opus preclarum anathomie totius corporis humani*. This section is at the end of the book and has separate pagination.

44. Si foetus mas fuerit, & per aborsum in dies quadraginta excidat: aperta matrice, cum humore super terram exiens a vulva dissolvetur sua teneritudine, & non invenietur propter sui parvitatem: si autem aborsus fuerit super aquam frigidam, levem & claram, invenietur per colamentum creatura, & habebit formam magnae formicae. Zerbi, "De generatione embrionis" in *Opus preclarum anathomie totius corporis humani*, fol. 14v.

45. Et aliquando quando recenter scinditur, invenitur habens motum dilationis & constrictionis quando acu pungitur, propter quod vere scitur creaturam illam esse animatam & invenitur quod veretrum eius & oculi eius magna sunt respectu suae quantitatis, eo que adhuc non sunt completa & adunata, sed in materia fluida resultat forma & figura membrorum, & simile evenit in aliis animalibus in oculis & membro generationis, ante ultimum eorum complementum, semper enim membra haec aliorum respectu magnam habent quantitatem. Zerbi, "De generatione embrionis" in *Opus preclarum anathomie totius corporis humani*, fol. 14v.

46. Colombo, *De re anatomica*, 245–252. For biographical information on Colombo, see Cunningham, "Columbus: The Revival of Alexandrian Anatomy," chap. 5 in *The Anatomical Renaissance*; On Colombo's discussion of fetal development, see also Berns, *The Bible and Natural Philosophy in Renaissance Italy*, 187–92. Some of my translations of Realdo Colombo's text follow Berns's translations.

47. quae in brutis imperfecte observabant, ad hominem maximo errore transtulerant, Colombo, *De re anatomica*, 246.

48. magnus Hippocrates, qui omnia scire non potuit solus, Colombo, *De re anatomica*, 249.

49. In canibus haec, quam dicimus, secundina est instar fasciae, quemadmodum illam Vessalius pinxit, qui caninam pro humana pinxit; licet in ea non catellum, sed infantulum pinxerit; sed secundina in homine est, quemadmodum ego supra explicavi. Colombo, *De re anatomica*, 248.

50. quemadmodum mihi non semel, sed saepius intueri, & animadvertere contigit. Colombo, *De re anatomica*, 247.

51. Hanc veritatem corona illustrium virorum, & praeccelentium magna cum voluptate vidit in Romano theatro: cum Hieronymus Pontanus summus Philosophus embrionem menstruum mihi publice dissecandum tradidisset, ob communem Romanae Academiae utilitatem: reliquorum autem membrorum quod primo fiat, quod posterius,

nondum mihi licuit observare: cum abortuum non ea sit copia, quae in tanta re necessaria esset. Colombo, *De re anatomica*, 247.

52. Coiter, "Ossium tum humani foetus adhuc in utero existentis, vel imperfecti abortus, tum infantis dimidium annum nati brevis historia atque explicatio" in *Externarum et Internarum Principalium*, 57–62.

53. Deinde his de causis ante multos annos puerorum Scheleta Bononiae mihi paravi, eorum vero ossa in scholis cum adultorum ossibus contuli & differentiam eorum auditoribus, tum explicavi, tum demonstravi. Coiter, "Ossium tum humani foetus," 57.

54. Talem & ego Bononiae in aedibus Doctoris Arantii vidi: porro Fernelius, caput par erat avellanae, & maius quam pro reliqui corporis ratione: oculi ut cancris exerti: nasus, auriculae, brachia, manus, crura, pedes, hisque secreti digiti: penis conspicuus, sub quo scrotum milii magnitudine, superiora inferioribus maiora, nullo ossium robore, sed flexibilia quocunque ducerentur. Coiter, "Ossium tum humani foetus," 58.

55. Porro equidem in meis aedibus Bononiae demonstravi abortum, qui digiti longitudinem habebat, hominisque integri figuram undequaque exprimebat. deprehendi conspicue admodum ossa bregmatis, ossa syncipitis & occipitis pro temporis ratitione [sic] admodum mollia. Coiter, "Ossium tum humani foetus," 59.

56. Hansen, "Resurrecting Death," 663–679.

57. Margócsy, "Advertising Cadavers," 188

58. Margócsy, "Advertising Cadavers," 197.

59. Knoeff, "Touching Anatomy," 35.

60. Knoeff, "Touching Anatomy."

61. Hansen, "Resurrecting Death."

62. Knoeff, "Touching Anatomy," 42–43.

63. Margócsy, "Advertising Cadavers," 205

64. Kunstkamera, "Collection Online."

65. Knoeff, "Touching Anatomy."

66. Knox, *The Anatomist's Instructor*.

67. Kaufman, "Frederick Knox," 44–56.

68. Knox, *The Anatomist's Instructor*, 132.

69. Hopwood, "Producing Development," 38 and 39.

70. On Mall, see Morgan, *Icons of Life*; Withycombe, *Lost*, 129–130, and Dubow, *Ourselves Unborn*, 14–15.

71. Withycombe, *Lost*, 127.

72. Withycombe, *Lost*.

73. Kenny, "The Development of Medical Museums," 32–62.

74. Morgan, *Icons of Life*, 125–133, quote on p. 129.

75. Chicago Museum of Science and Industry, "Prenatal Development."

76. Dubow, *Ourselves Unborn*, 39–40, quote p. 40.

77. Chicago Museum of Science and Industry, "Prenatal Development."

78. Dubow, *Ourselves Unborn*, 41.

79. Petchesky, "Fetal Images," 268.

80. This is the definition used by the World Health Organization. The Centers for Disease Control and Prevention definition includes deaths up to a year after the end of the pregnancy. Centers for Disease Control and Prevention, "Maternal Mortality."

81. Tikkanen et al., "Maternal Mortality and Maternity Care."

82. D'Alton, "Where Is the 'M' in Maternal–Fetal Medicine?," 1401–1404; Martin and Montagne, "The Last Person You'd Expect to Die in Childbirth"; MacDorman et al., "Recent Increases in the U.S. Maternal Mortality Rate," 447–455.

83. Dembosky, "Health Department Medical Detectives."

84. Martin and Montagne, "The Last Person You'd Expect to Die in Childbirth."

85. D'Alton, "Where Is the 'M' in Maternal–Fetal Medicine?," 1401–1404.

86. D'Alton et al., "Putting the 'M' Back in Maternal-Fetal Medicine," 311–317.

87. Grimes, "The Morbidity and Mortality of Pregnancy," 1489–1494.

88. Centers for Disease Control, "Maternal and Infant Health."

89. Cheng, Fowles, and Walker, "Postpartum Maternal Health Care," 34–42.

90. Cheng, Fowles, and Walker, "Postpartum Maternal Health Care."

91. Haertsch, "After Birth."

92. Francis, Cheung, and Berger, "How Does the U.S. Compare."

93. Martin and Montagne, "Nothing Protects Black Women." See also Tucker et al., "The Black-White Disparity." 247–251.

94. Martin and Montagne, "Nothing Protects Black Women."

95. Martin and Montagne, "Nothing Protects Black Women."

96. Wailoo, "The Pain Gap."

97. Centers for Disease Control, "Folic Acid."

98. Casper, *Babylost*, 102–104, quote on p. 103.

99. Commonwealth Fund, "Policies for Reducing Maternal Morbidity and Mortality."

3   THE DANGEROUS WOMB

1. Goldberg, "When a Miscarriage Is Manslaughter"; Tsai, "Why We Can't Look Away"; McClung and Bailey, "She Was Charged with Manslaughter after a Miscarriage."
2. Ava B., "When Miscarriage Is a Crime."
3. Kuriyama, *The Expressiveness of the Body*, esp. chap. 3.
4. On ancient gynecology, see King, *Hippocrates' Woman*.
5. Aristotle, *Generation of Animals*, 95.
6. Aristotle, *Generation of Animals*, 101. Emphasis in original.
7. Aristotle, *Generation of Animals*, 119.
8. Aristotle, *Generation of Animals*, 103.
9. Lonie, *The Hippocratic Treatises*, 2.
10. Lonie, *The Hippocratic Treatises*, 7.
11. Lonie, *The Hippocratic Treatises*, 8.
12. Lonie, *The Hippocratic Treatises*, 8.
13. For more on this topic, see Dean-Jones, "Menstrual Bleeding According to the Hippocratics and Aristotle," 177–191.
14. *Soranus' Gynecology*, 34.
15. *Soranus' Gynecology*, 23.
16. On medieval obstetrics and gynecology, see Cadden, *Meanings of Sex Difference* and Green, *Making Women's Medicine Masculine*.
17. Lemay, *Women's Secrets*, 63.
18. Lemay, *Women's Secrets*, 60.
19. Crawford, "Attitudes to Menstruation in Seventeenth-Century England," 47–73; McClive, *Menstruation and Procreation in Early Modern France*; Read, *Menstruation and the Female Body in Early Modern England*.
20. Sędziwój, *A New Light of Alchymie*.
21. Greenhill, *A Treatise on the Small-Pox and Measles*.
22. Avicenna, *Canon medicinae*, 72–76.
23. Siraisi, *Avicenna in Renaissance Italy*.
24. "Variola eminentiam facit accidit autem hec species frequentius pueris generatur tempore menstruorum vel nutricis in utero menstruali sangue non von depurato." Gilbertus Anglicus (Gilbert the Englishman), *Compendium medicine*, fol. cccxlvii.
25. "Ista passio generatur ex sangunie menstruo retento in porositatibus membrorum fetorum." Bernardus de Gordonio (Gordonius; Bernard de Gordon), *Practica seu Lilium medicine*, unpag. 15 verso.

26. "ex corruptione sanginis menstrui pervenientia." Johannes de Gaddesden (John of Gaddesden), *Rosa anglica practica medicine a capite ad pedes*, fol. 40 verso.

27. "nam ex puriori parte fetus nutritur feculentia autem in porositatibus retinetur." Valesco de Tarenta, *Practica valesci de tharanta que alias philonium dicitur*, fol. 242 recto.

28. Kellwaye, *A Defensatiue against the*, cap. i, fol. 39 recto.

29. van Diemerbroeck, *The Anatomy of Human Bodies*, chap. 3, pp. 4–7.

30. Westwood, *De variolis & morbillis*, 7–9.

31. Genesis 30:37–38.

32. Aetius (c. 90 AD), Fragment 5.12.2 (Dox. Gr. 423), quoted in Inwood, *The Poem of Empedocles*, 185.

33. *Soranus' Gynecology*, 37–38.

34. Rublack, "Pregnancy, Childbirth and the Female Body," 84–110.

35. Paré, *On Monsters and Marvels*, 38–42.

36. Weingarten, "What to Expect When You're Expecting in the Nineteenth-Century U.S."

37. Pancoast, *Ladies' Medical Guide*, 200.

38. Napheys, *The Physical Life of Woman*, 115–116.

39. Musacchio, *The Art and Ritual of Childbirth*.

40. Buonarroti, *Holy Family*.

41. Pancoast, *Ladies' Medical Guide*, 208.

42. Napheys, *The Physical Life of Woman*, 115–116.

43. *Soranus' Gynecology*, 47.

44. *Soranus' Gynecology*, 48.

45. *Soranus' Gynecology*, 49–50.

46. *Soranus' Gynecology*, 53–54.

47. *Soranus' Gynecology*, 55.

48. *Soranus' Gynecology*, 80.

49. Avicenna, *Canon medicinae*.

50. Marafioti, "The Prescriptive Potency of Food," 28. See also Savonarola, *Il trattato ginecologico-pediatrico in volgare*.

51. Marafioti, "The Prescriptive Potency of Food," 19–33.

52. West, *Prenatal Care*, 8.

53. West, *Prenatal Care*, 11.

54. Benjamin, Fee, and Brown, "William Augustus Evans (1865–1948)," 2073.

55. Evans, "How to Keep Well," 12.

56. Eisenberg, Murkoff and Hathaway, *What to Expect When You're Expecting*, 80.

57. Eisenberg, Murkoff, and Hathaway, *What to Expect When You're Expecting*, 80.
58. Eisenberg, Murkoff, and Hathaway, *What to Expect When You're Expecting*, 81.
59. Corriente, *Dictionary of Arabic and Allied Loanwords*, definitions on pp. 54 and 478, respectively.
60. Tomes, *The Gospel of Germs*.
61. Eisenberg, Murkoff, and Hathaway, *What to Expect When You're Expecting*, 184.
62. Oster, *Expecting Better*.
63. Werber, "The 'Dos' and 'Don'ts' of Pregnancy Are Deeply Flawed."
64. Shaw, "Chicken of the Sea."
65. Payer, *Medicine and Culture*.
66. Bonnell Freidin, "Well-Born."
67. Quoted in Marafioti, "The Prescriptive Potency of Food," 30.
68. Eisenberg, Murkoff, and Hathaway, *What to Expect When You're Expecting*, 94–95.
69. Eisenberg, Murkoff, and Hathaway, *What to Expect When You're Expecting*, 128.
70. Monsivais and Drewnowski, "The Rising Cost of Low-Energy-Density Foods," 2071–2076.
71. Monsivais and Drewnowski, "Lower-Energy-Density Diets Are Associated with Higher Monetary Costs," 814–822; Brown et al., "Food Insecurity and Obesity," 980–987.
72. Integris Health, "What Is a Food Desert?"
73. Raglan et al., "Racial and Ethnic Disparities," 16–24; Heck et al., "Maternal Mortality among American Indian / Alaska Native Women"; Gurr, "Complex Intersections," 721–735.
74. US Census Bureau, "Comanche County, Oklahoma," QuickFacts, https://www.census.gov/quickfacts/fact/table/comanchecounty oklahoma/PST045219. See also "Oklahoma State Department of Health State of the County's Health Report, Comanche County, Summer 2017," https://oklahoma.gov/health/community-health /community-epidemiology/county-health-profiles.html, and Oklahoma State Board of Health, "State of the State's Health," https:// stateofstateshealth.ok.gov/.
75. Oklahoma State Board of Health, "State of the State's Health."
76. LaVarnway and Craven, "An Overview of Food Deserts in Oklahoma."

77. McClung, "Oklahoma Completes First-Ever Report on Maternal Deaths."
78. Maternal Vulnerability Index.
79. New York Times Editorial Board, "Slandering the Unborn."
80. Flavin, *Our Bodies, Our Crimes*, 107.
81. Flavin, *Our Bodies, Our Crimes*, 108.
82. Martin, "Take a Valium, Lose Your Kid, Go to Jail."
83. Flavin, *Our Bodies, Our Crimes*, 105. See also Martin, "Take a Valium, Lose Your Kid, Go to Jail."
84. Quoted in Morgan, *Icons of Life*, 54.
85. West, *Prenatal Care*, 19.
86. Quoted in Morgan, *Icons of Life*, 53.
87. Brady, "Are Babies 'Marked' By Prenatal Influence?"
88. S. P. Sackett, *Mother, Nurse, and Infant: A Manual* (New York: H. Campbell Co., 1889), p. 21. Quoted in Weingarten, "What to Expect When You're Expecting in the Nineteenth-Century U.S."
89. West, *Prenatal Care*, 20.
90. Reed, *What Every Expectant Mother Should Know*, 16.
91. Fatima, Srivastav, and Mondal, "Prenatal Stress and Depression," 1–7; Lazinski, Shea, and Steiner, "Effects of Maternal Prenatal Stress," 363–375; Nowak et al., "Stress during Pregnancy and Epigenetic Modifications," 134–145; Chahal et al., "Relation of Outbursts of Anger and the Acute Risk of Placental Abruption," 405–411.
92. Cep, "The Perils and Possibilities of Anger"; Harris-Perry, *Sister Citizen*.
93. Pearlin, "The Sociological Study of Stress," 241–256.
94. Duden, *The Woman beneath the Skin*, 141–142.
95. Stockman "Manslaughter Charge Dropped."
96. Abouk and Adams, "Birth Outcomes in Flint," 68–85.
97. Grossman and Slusky, "The Impact of the Flint Water Crisis on Fertility," 2005–2031.
98. Edwards, "Fetal Death and Reduced Birth Rates," 739–746.
99. Grossman and Slusky, "The Impact of the Flint Water Crisis on Fertility."
100. Lewis, Hoover, and MacKenzie, "Mining and Environmental Health Disparities," 130–141. See also Agency for Toxic Substances and Disease Registry (ATSDR), "Navajo Birth Cohort Study," https://www.atsdr.cdc.gov/sites/navajo_birth_cohort_study/index.html.
101. UC Berkeley, "CHAMACOS Study."
102. Hall, "The Lost Generation."
103. Casper, *Babylost*, 65–69.

4 THE SECRETS OF WOMEN

1. Phillip, "Mark Zuckerberg and Priscilla Chan's Refreshingly Honest Facebook Post"; Haelle, "Zuckerberg Helps Destigmatize Miscarriage"; Abbott and Declercq, "Zuckerberg's Important Message on Miscarriage."
2. Zauzmer, "Pregnant Carrie Underwood."
3. Fisher and Underwood, "I Am Second."
4. Rubenstein, "Inside Carrie Underwood's Emotional Journey."
5. McKnight, "How Carrie Underwood Dealt with Three Heartbreaking Miscarriages."
6. Meghan, The Duchess of Sussex, "The Losses We Share."
7. Withycombe, *Lost*, 162.
8. Withycombe, *Lost*, 162.
9. Withycombe, *Lost*, 163. See also Grose, "After a Miscarriage."
10. Goldberg, "When a Miscarriage Is Manslaughter."
11. Freidenfelds, *The Myth of the Perfect Pregnancy*; Withycombe, *Lost*.
12. Freidenfelds, *The Myth of the Perfect Pregnancy*.
13. Lemay, *Women's Secrets*, 59.
14. Park, *Secrets of Women*.
15. Park, *Secrets of Women*, 96. See also Green, *Making Women's Medicine Masculine*.
16. Lemay, *Women's Secrets*, 88.
17. Lemay, *Women's Secrets*, 120.
18. Lemay, *Women's Secrets*, 121.
19. Lemay, *Women's Secrets*, 65.
20. Lemay, *Women's Secrets*, 102. But I follow Park's translation of this passage. Park, *Secrets of Women*, 84.
21. Lemay, *Women's Secrets*, 125.
22. Hippocrates of Cos, *Nature of the Child*, in Lonie, *The Hippocratic Treatises*, 35.
23. *Soranus' Gynecology*, 43–44.
24. Guillemeau, *Child-birth*, 3–4
25. Sharp, *The Midwives Book*, 102–103.
26. *Aristoteles Master-piece*, 43.
27. Cadden, *Meanings of Sex Difference in the Middle Ages*, 150–154.
28. Hirst, *A Text-book of Obstetrics*, 71.
29. Edgar, *The Practice of Obstetrics*, 12.
30. Murkoff, *What to Expect When You're Expecting*.
31. Tucker, "The Medieval Roots of Todd Akin's Theories."

32. Receipt book, 58.

33. *Aristoteles Master-piece*, 43.

34. Guillemeau, *Child-birth*, 6.

35. On the importance of recipe books in the early modern period, see Leong, *Recipes and Everyday Knowledge*.

36. Boyle Family, recipe book, fol. 16v.

37. Receipt book, 58.

38. Sheppey, A Book of Choice Receipts, 454.

39. *Soranus' Gynecology*, 45–46.

40. Guillemeau, *Child-birth*, 22.

41. Sharp, *The Midwives Book*, 224.

42. *Aristoteles Master-piece*, 47.

43. Freidenfelds, *The Myth of the Perfect Pregnancy*, 22.

44. Duden, *Woman beneath the Skin*, 142.

45. *Soranus' Gynecology*, 66.

46. Lemay, *Secrets of Women*, 79.

47. *Aristoteles Master-piece*, 47.

48. Sharp, *The Midwives Book*, 224–5.

49. Boyle Family, recipe book, fol. 104v, #407.

50. Sheppey, A Book of Choice Receipts, 450.

51. Drake, "The Eagle Stone," 128–132, references to Pliny on pp. 128–130.

52. Dols, "The Origins of the Islamic Hospital," 378.

53. Strocchia, *Forgotten Healers*, 74.

54. Fissell, "The Politics of Reproduction in the English Reformation," 44.

55. Duden, *Woman Beneath the Skin*, 159.

56. Freidenfelds, *The Myth of the Perfect Pregnancy*; Withycombe, *Lost*; McClive, *Menstruation and Procreation*.

57. Arenfeldt, "The Political Role of the Female Consort," 220–223.

58. Arenfeldt, "The Political Role of the Female Consort," 203–213.

59. McClive, *Menstruation and Procreation*, 118.

60. McClive, *Menstruation and Procreation*, 140.

61. Harkness, "Managing an Experimental Household," 256.

62. Wikisource, "Diary of Samuel Pepys/1660/January," https://en.wiki source.org/wiki/Diary_of_Samuel_Pepys/1660/January.

63. Duden, *Woman Beneath the Skin*, 146–147, quotes on p. 147.

64. McClive, *Menstruation and Procreation*, 119–120.

65. Kassell, "Fruitful Bodies and Astrological Medicine," 224–240, esp. 230–235.

66. Kassell et al., *The Casebooks of Simon Forman and Richard Napier*.

67. Kassell et al., *The Casebooks of Simon Forman and Richard Napier*.
68. Kassell et al., *The Casebooks of Simon Forman and Richard Napier*.
69. Sharp, *The Midwives Book*, 103.
70. List drawn from Sharp, *The Midwives Book*; *Soranus' Gynecology*; Guillemeau *Child-birth*; and *Aristoteles Master-piece*.
71. Quoted in Arenfeldt, "The Political Role of the Female Consort," 209.
72. Duden, *Woman Beneath the Skin*, 111.
73. McClive, *Menstruation and Procreation*, 152.
74. Arenfeldt, "The Political Role of the Female Consort," 215.
75. Duden, *Woman Beneath the Skin*, 160.
76. Duden, *Woman Beneath the Skin*, 161.
77. McClive, *Menstruation and Procreation*, 218.
78. Poppick, "The Long, Winding Tale of Sperm Science,"
79. Luthra and Johnston, "Texas' Governor Got a Basic Fact about Pregnancy Wrong."
80. Jarvis, "Early Embryo Mortality in Natural Human Reproduction"; Jarvis, "Misjudging Early Embryo Mortality in Natural Human Reproduction."
81. Wilcox et al., "Incidence of Early Loss of Pregnancy," 189–194; Zinaman et al., "Estimates of Human Fertility and Pregnancy Loss," 503–509.
82. Cohain, Buxbaum, and Mankuta, "Spontaneous First Trimester Miscarriage Rates."
83. American College of Obstetricians and Gynecologists, "Early Pregnancy Loss"; see similar advice in Mayo Clinic, "Miscarriage," and Gelman, "4 Things That Can Cause a Miscarriage."
84. Bardos et al., "A National Survey on Public Perceptions of Miscarriage," 1313–1320. Study discussed in Withycombe, *Lost*.
85. Riggs et al., "Men, Trans/Masculine, and Non-Binary People's Experiences of Pregnancy Loss."
86. Schaffir, "Do Patients Associate Adverse Pregnancy Outcomes with Folkloric Beliefs?"
87. Schaffir, "Do Patients Associate Adverse Pregnancy Outcomes with Folkloric Beliefs?," 301.
88. Freidenfelds, *The Myth of the Perfect Pregnancy*, 191.
89. Pilkington, "Murder Charges Dropped against Texas Woman."
90. Quoted in Martinez, "Latinx Files."
91. Casper, *Babylost*, 20.
92. Fractracker Alliance, "Oklahoma," https://www.fractracker.org/map/us/oklahoma/.

93. Apergis, Hayat, and Saeed, "Fracking and Infant Mortality."
94. Casper, *Babylost*, 20, emphasis in original.
95. Brown, "Mom Brings Miscarried Fetus to City Council Meeting." Daniela Blei discusses Taylor's story in "The History of Talking about Miscarriage."

5 ABORTION AND THE FETUS

1. Holland, *Tiny You*; Mohr, *Abortion in America*; Reagan, *When Abortion Was a Crime*; Solinger, *Abortion Wars*.
2. *Roe v. Wade*.
3. *Dobbs v. Jackson Women's Health Organization*.
4. *Roe v. Wade*.
5. Mulder, "The Hippocratic Oath in *Roe v. Wade*."
6. Hasday, "On Roe, Alito Cites a Judge Who Treated Women as Witches and Property."
7. Hippocrates, *Nature of the Child*, 35–37.
8. Kapparis, *Abortion in the Ancient World*, 98.
9. Feen, "The Historical Dimensions of Infanticide and Abortion." See also Gardner, *Women in Roman Law and Society*.
10. Mulder, "Ancient Medicine and Fetal Personhood."
11. Cicero, *Pro Lege Manilia*, 255. Quoted in Mulder, "Ancient Medicine and Fetal Personhood." See also Kapparis, *Abortion in the Ancient World*, 138, 193–194, and Mistry, *Abortion in the Early Middle Ages*, 25–28.
12. Mulder, "Ancient Medicine and Fetal Personhood." Mulder cites Aulus Gellius, Tacitus, and Juvenal. I have used the same quotes but from the Loeb translations. See also Kapparis, *Abortion in the Ancient World*, 97–120 and 148–150, and Mistry, *Abortion in the Early Middle Ages*, 32–34.
13. Pliny, *Natural History*, vol. 3, bk 10, p. 401.
14. Tacitus, *Annals*, 209
15. Gellius, *Attic Nights*, 1:355.
16. Juvenal, *Juvenal and Persius*, 289. See also Kapparis, *Abortion in the Ancient World*, 83.
17. The Latin reads, "homines in ventre necandos." Juvenal, *Juvenal and Persius*, 288.
18. *Soranus' Gynecology*, 62–68. Quotes on p. 63.
19. Aristotle, *Politics*, 623–625. See also Lu, "Aristotle on Abortion and Infanticide," 47–62.
20. Kapparis, "The Man's Point of View," chapter 5 in *Abortion in the Ancient World*.

21. Roberts, *Killing the Black Body*, 41.
22. Bush-Slimani, "Hard Labour," 83–99, esp. 92; Roberts, *Killing the Black Body*, 39–55.
23. Roberts, *Killing the Black Body*, 46–47.
24. Karol K. Weaver, "'She Crushed the Child's Fragile Skull,'" 93–109, quote on p. 99.
25. From the *Vita sancti Ciarani episcopi Saigirensis*. Quoted in Callan, "Of Vanishing Fetuses and Maidens Made-Again," 290. See also Mistry, "The Sexual Shame of the Chaste."
26. Callan, "Of Vanishing Fetuses and Maidens Made-Again," 290.
27. Callan, "Of Vanishing Fetuses and Maidens Made-Again," 292.
28. Callan, "Of Vanishing Fetuses and Maidens Made-Again," 295.
29. Callan, "Saints Once Did Abortions."
30. Salés, "As Texas Ban on Abortion Goes into Effect."
31. United States Conference of Catholic Bishops, "Respect for Unborn Human Life." My emphasis.
32. Abolish Human Abortion, "Abolitionism through the Ages," https://abolishhumanabortion.com/what-is-an-abolitionist/.
33. On similarities between Roman pagan and Christian views on abortion, see Mistry, *Abortion in the Early Middle Ages*.
34. Lemay, *Women's Secrets*, 79.
35. Lemay, *Women's Secrets*, 103.
36. Chrysostom, "Homily 24 on Romans."
37. Green, "Constantinus Africanus," 47–69, 54–60.
38. Green, "Constantinus Africanus," 48–50.
39. For spelling of his name, death date, and translation of the Arabic title of his book, I follow Zaimeche, "Ibn al-Jazzār."
40. Green, "Constantinus Africanus," 50.
41. Green, "Constantinus Africanus," 52–53, quote on p. 53.
42. Green, "Constantinus Africanus," 53.
43. Scarborough, "Theodora, Aetius of Amida, and Procopius," 742–762, list of abortifacient substances on p. 753.
44. Gurunluoglu and Gurunluoglu, "Paul of Aegina."
45. Hoberock, "Oklahoma Senate Passes Three Controversial Bills."
46. Wilcox, "Poisoning by Pennyroyal," 394. This case is cited in Wierzbicki, "A Cup of Pennyroyal Tea."
47. Mohr, *Abortion in America*, 25–26.
48. Mohr, *Abortion in America*, 86.
49. Roosevelt, "On American Motherhood."

50. Freidenfelds, *The Myth of the Perfect Pregnancy*, esp. chaps. 1 and 2. On fertility rates and pregnancy in the eighteenth century, see also Leavitt, *Brought to Bed*.

51. Mohr, *Abortion in America*.

52. Kapparis, "Methods of Abortion: Science and Superstition," chap. 1 in *Abortion in the Ancient World*.

53. Totelin, "Sex and Vegetables," 536.

54. King, "Hippocrates Didn't Write the Oath." See also Kapparis, *Abortion in the Ancient World*, 66–76.

55. Dioscorides, *De materia medica*, 324.

56. Dioscorides, *De materia medica*, 423.

57. Dioscorides, *De materia medica*, 404.

58. Dioscorides, *De materia medica*, 513.

59. Dioscorides, *De materia medica*, 412.

60. Pliny, *Natural History*, vol. 6, bk 20, p. 131.

61. Pliny, *Natural History*, vol. 6, bk 20, p. 145.

62. Pliny. *Natural History*, vol. 6, bk 20 p. 9.

63. *Soranus' Gynecology*, 62–68, quotes on p. 63.

64. van de Walle, "Flowers and Fruits," 192.

65. van de Walle, "Flowers and Fruits," 192–193.

66. Gerard, *The Herball*, 672.

67. Gerard, *The Herball*, 1257.

68. Riddle, *Eve's Herbs*, 40–63.

69. Dickson, "Herbal Abortions Are Going Viral on TikTok"; Lucas, "Dangerous Herbal Abortion Misinformation."

70. Amazon, "*What to Expect When You're Expecting*, Kindle Edition," accessed August 31, 2022, https://www.amazon.com/What-Expect-When-Youre-Expecting-ebook/dp/B01DCHZE3A/ref=tmm_kin_swatch_0?_encoding=UTF8&qid=1661964715&sr=8–1.

71. Quoted in Kapparis, *Abortion in the Ancient World*, 16.

72. Kapparis, *Abortion in the Ancient World*, 195.

73. Lucas, "Dangerous Herbal Abortion Misinformation."

74. van de Walle, "Flowers and Fruits," 203.

75. Quoted in Sweet, "Hildegard of Bingen and the Greening of Medieval Medicine," 381–403.

76. Riddle, *Eve's Herbs*, 58–59.

77. Riddle, *Eve's Herbs*, 47; Totelin, "Sex and Vegetables," 536.

78. Totelin, "Sex and Vegetables," 536.

79. Totelin, "Sex and Vegetables," 536.

80. Bacon, receipt book, 254.

81. Bacon, receipt book.

82. Riddle, *Eve's Herbs*, 56.

83. I owe this point to Freidenfelds, "The Historical Creation and Implications of the Distinction between Miscarriage and Abortion."

84. Freedman, Landy, and Steinauer, "When There's a Heartbeat."

85. Specia, "How Savita Halappanavar's Death Spurred Ireland's Abortion Rights Campaign"; Holland, "How the Death of Savita Halappanavar Revolutionised Ireland."

86. Sellers and Nirappil, "Confusion Post-*Roe* Spurs Delays."

87. See for example Mendola, "Rivers of Babylon," and Waldman, "On Feeling Like a 'Bad Mother.'" Whole Woman's Health invites people to share their abortion stories at https://www.wholewomanshealth.com/share-your-abortion-story/.

CONCLUSION

1. McCulloch, "The Rise of the Fetal Citizen," 20.

2. Alexandria Ocasio-Cortez (@AOC), Twitter, May 8, 2019, 12:28 a.m., https://twitter.com/AOC/status/1125980728976715776.

3. Liz Wheeler (@Liz_Wheeler), Twitter, May 8, 2019, 10:57 a.m., https://twitter.com/Liz_Wheeler/status/1126138964346150914.

4. In physicist Erwin Schrödinger's thought experiment, a cat is placed in a sealed box with a container of poison, a quantity of radioactive material, and a Geiger counter to measure the radiation. As soon as a single atom of the radioactive material decays, it sets off the Geiger counter, which shatters the container of poison and kills the cat. But the experimenter does not know how long it will take for the radioactive decay to occur that will trigger the release of the poison and the death of the cat. Looking at the sealed box from the outside, he or she cannot know whether the cat is alive or dead. Rather, the possibilities of live and dead cat exist simultaneously in the box until it is opened.

5. Shepherd and Sellers, "Abortion Bans Complicate Access to Drugs for Cancer, Arthritis, Even Ulcers"; Sharp, "Post-*Roe*, Many Autoimmune Patients Lose Access to 'Gold Standard' Drug."

6. "Abortion Ban May Mean Denial of Effective Drugs for Women with MS, Migraine, Epilepsy."

7. Christian and Borges, "What *Dobbs* Means for Patients with Breast Cancer."

8. Fissell, "The Politics of Reproduction in the English Reformation," 58–59.

BIBLIOGRAPHY

Abbott, Jodi F., and Eugene Declercq. "Zuckerberg's Important Message on Miscarriage." CNN, August 5, 2015. https://www.cnn.com/2015/08/05/opinions/abbott-declercq-pregnancy-loss/index.html.

Abolish Human Abortion. https://abolishhumanabortion.com/.

"Abortion Ban May Mean Denial of Effective Drugs for Women with MS, Migraine, Epilepsy: Perspective Article Says New Ruling May Result in Increased Risk of Deaths, Disability." *Science Daily*, July 13, 2022. https://www.sciencedaily.com/releases/2022/07/220713163355.htm.

Abouk, Rahi, and Scott Adams. "Birth Outcomes in Flint in the Early Stages of the Water Crisis." *Journal of Public Health Policy* 39 (2018): 68–85.

American College of Obstetricians and Gynecologists. "Early Pregnancy Loss: Frequently Asked Questions." https://www.acog.org/womens-health/faqs/early-pregnancy-loss.

Apergis, Nicholas, Tasawar Hayat, and Tareq Saeed. "Fracking and Infant Mortality: Fresh Evidence from Oklahoma." *Environmental Science and Pollution Research* 26 (2019): 32360–32367.

Arenfeldt, Pernille. "The Political Role of the Female Consort in Protestant Germany, 1550–1585: Anna of Saxony as *Mater Patriae*." PhD thesis, Florence, European University Institute, Department of History and Civilization, 2006. http://hdl.handle.net/1814/5815.

Aristotle. *Generation of Animals*. Translated by A. L. Peck. Loeb Classical Library 366. Cambridge, MA: Harvard University Press, 1942.

Aristotle. *History of Animals.* Vol. 3, bks 7–10. Edited and translated by
 D. M. Balme. Loeb Classical Library 439. Cambridge, MA: Harvard
 University Press, 1991.

Aristotle. *On the Parts of Animals.* Translated by William Ogle, bk 3, part 4.
 http://classics.mit.edu/Aristotle/parts_animals.3.iii.html.

Aristotle. *On the Soul. Parva Naturalia. On Breath.* Translated by W. S. Hett.
 Loeb Classical Library 288. Cambridge, MA: Harvard University
 Press, 1957.

Aristotle. *Parts of Animals. Movement of Animals. Progression of Animals.*
 Translated by A. L. Peck and E. S. Forster. Loeb Classical Library 323.
 Cambridge, MA: Harvard University Press, 1937.

Aristotle. *Politics.* Translated by H. Rackham. Loeb Classical Library 264.
 Cambridge, MA: Harvard University Press, 1932.

*Aristotele's Master-piece, or The Secrets of Generation Displayed in All the
 Parts Thereof.* London: J. How, 1684.

Armstrong, Elizabeth M. *Conceiving Risk, Bearing Responsibility: Fetal
 Alcohol Syndrome and the Diagnosis of Moral Disorder.* Baltimore:
 Johns Hopkins University Press, 2003.

Aspinwall, Cary, Brianna Bailey, and Amy Yurkanin. "They Lost Pregnancies for Unclear Reasons. Then They Were Prosecuted." *Washington
 Post,* September 12, 2022. https://www.washingtonpost.com/national
 -security/2022/09/01/prosecutions-drugs-miscarriages-meth-stillbirths/.

Augustine. *The Confessions of Saint Augustine.* Translated by E. B. Pusey.
 N.p.: Project Gutenberg, 2002. https://www.gutenberg.org/files/3296
 /3296-h/3296-h.htm.

Avicenna. *Canon medicinae.* Venice: Junta, 1595.

B., Ava. "When Miscarriage Is a Crime." *Planned Parenthood Advocates of
 Arizona* (blog), July 29, 2019. https://www.plannedparenthoodaction
 .org/planned-parenthood-advocates-arizona/blog/when-miscarriage
 -is-a-crime.

Bacon, Catherine. Receipt book. Unpublished manuscript, c. 1680–1739.
 Folger Shakespeare Library. https://luna.folger.edu/luna/servlet (call
 no. v.a.621 [332]).

Bardos, Jonah, Daniel Hercz, Jenna Friedenthal, Stacey A. Missmer, and
 Zev Williams. "A National Survey on Public Perceptions of Miscarriage." *Obstetrics and Gynecology* 125, no. 6 (2015): 1313–1320. https://doi
 .org/0.1097/AOG.0000000000000859.

Bates, Laura. *Everyday Sexism.* London: Simon and Schuster, 2014.

Bauhin, Caspar. *Theatrum anatomicum / novis figuris aeneis illustratum, et in lucem emissum opera et sumptibus Theodori de Bry*. Frankfurt: M. Becker, 1605.

Benjamin, Georges C., Elizabeth Fee, and Theodore M. Brown. "William Augustus Evans (1865–1948): Public Health Leader at a Critical Time." *American Journal of Public Health* 100, no. 11 (2010): 2073.

Berger, Margret. *Hildegard of Bingen: On Natural Philosophy and Medicine*. Selections from *Cause et cure*. Translated from Latin with introduction, notes, and interpretive essay. Rochester, NY: D. S. Brewer, 1999.

Bernardus de Gordonio (Gordonius; Bernard de Gordon). *Practica seu Lilium medicine*. Venice: Bonetus Locatellus, 1496/97.

Berns, Andrew D. *The Bible and Natural Philosophy in Renaissance Italy: Jewish and Christian Physicians in Search of Truth*. Cambridge: Cambridge University Press, 2014.

Blei, Daniela. "The History of Talking about Miscarriage." *The Cut*, April 23, 2018. https://www.thecut.com/2018/04/the-history-of-talking -about-miscarriage.html.

Boboltz, Sara. "Madison Cawthorn Thinks Your Pregnancy Is a Polaroid or a Sunset or Something." *Huffpost*, December 4, 2021. https://www .huffpost.com/entry/madison-cawthorns-simplistic-abortion-analogy -misses-the-point_n_61ab8ba1e4b0ae9a42bd4c76.

Bonnell Freidin, Anna. "Well-Born: The Ancient History of Making the Best Babies." *Eidolon*, December 26, 2016. https://eidolon.pub/well -born-the-ancient-history-of-making-the-best-babies-e396e2c2d6b7.

The Book of Common Prayer—1549. http://justus.anglican.org/resources /bcp/1549/Communion_1549.htm.

Bouley, Bradford A. *Pious Postmortems: Anatomy, Sanctity, and the Catholic Church in Early Modern Europe*. Philadelphia: University of Pennsylvania Press, 2017.

Boyle, Marjorie O'Rourke. "Broken Hearts: The Violation of Biblical Law." *Journal of the American Academy of Religion* 73, no. 3 (September 2005): 731–757.

Boyle Family. Recipe book. c. 1675–c. 1710. Wellcome Collection. https:// wellcomecollection.org/works/hyf3jbn9.

Brady, William. "Are Babies 'Marked' by Prenatal Influence?" *Los Angeles Times*, June 26, 1932.

Brown, Alison G. M., Layla E. Esposito, Rachel A. Fisher, Holly L. Nicastro, Derrick C. Tabor, and Jenelle R. Walker. "Food Insecurity and Obesity:

Research Gaps, Opportunities, and Challenges." *Translational Behavioral Medicine* 9, no. 5 (October 2019): 980–987.

Brown, Shelby. "Mom Brings Miscarried Fetus to City Council Meeting, Calls for Change." Channel 6 News, Richmond, February 27, 2018. https://www.wtvr.com/2018/02/27/mom-brings-miscarried-fetus-to-city -council-meeting-calls-for-change.

Buonarroti, Michelangelo. *Holy Family, Known as the "Doni Tondo."* 1505–1506. Tempera grassa on wood. Florence, The Uffizi Gallery, inv. no. 1890 n. 1456. https://www.uffizi.it/en/artworks/holy-family-known -as-the-doni-tondo.

Bush-Slimani, Barbara. "Hard Labour: Women, Childbirth and Resistance in British Caribbean Slave Societies." *History Workshop Journal* 36 (1992): 83–99.

Buzzfeed. "23 Extremely Difficult Side Effects Of Pregnancy That No One Warns You About." November 17, 2021. https://www.buzzfeed.com /simrinsingh/harsh-side-effects-of-pregnancy.

Bylebyl, Jerome J. "Interpreting the 'Fasciculo' Anatomy Scene." *Journal of the History of Medicine and Allied Sciences* 45 (1990): 285–316.

Cadden, Joan. *Meanings of Sex Difference in the Middle Ages.* Cambridge: Cambridge University Press, 1993.

Callan, Maeve B. "Of Vanishing Fetuses and Maidens Made-Again: Abortion, Restored Virginity, and Similar Scenarios in Medieval Irish Hagiography and Penitentials." *Journal of the History of Sexuality* 21 (2012): 282–296.

Callan, Maeve B. "Saints Once Did Abortions—It Was a Lesser Sin than Oral Sex." *Irish Times*, April 19, 2018. https://www.irishtimes.com/culture /books/saints-once-did-abortions-it-was-a-lesser-sin-than-oral-sex-1 .3466881.

Calvin, John. *Institutes of the Christian Religion.* Grand Rapids, MI: William B. Eerdmans Publishing, 1995.

Carmon, Irin. "Fetus To 'Testify' In Support of Ohio Heartbeat Bill." Jezebel, March 1, 2011. https://jezebel.com/fetus-to-testify-in-support-of -ohio-heartbeat-bill-5773244.

Carmon, Irin. "Ohio Fetus Testimony Doesn't Go So Well." Jezebel, March 2, 2011. https://jezebel.com/ohio-fetus-testimony-doesnt-go-so -well-5774543.

"The Case of a Man, Whose Heart Was Found Enlarged to a Very Uncommon Size, by Mr. Richard Pulteney: Communicated by W. Watson, M.D. R.S.S." *Philosophical Transactions of the Royal Society* 52 (1761): 344–353.

Casper, Monica J. *Babylost: Racism, Survival, and the Quiet Politics of Infant Mortality, from A to Z*. New Brunswick, NJ: Rutgers University Press, 2022.

Casper, Monica J. *The Making of the Unborn Patient: A Social Anatomy of Fetal Surgery*. New Brunswick, NJ: Rutgers University Press, 1998.

Centers for Disease Control and Prevention. "Folic Acid." https://www.cdc.gov/ncbddd/folicacid/about.html.

Centers for Disease Control and Prevention. "Maternal and Infant Health." https://www.cdc.gov/reproductivehealth/maternalinfanthealth/.

Centers for Disease Control and Prevention. "Maternal Mortality." https://www.cdc.gov/reproductivehealth/maternal-mortality/index.html.

Cep, Casey. "The Perils and Possibilities of Anger: After Centuries of Censure, Women Reconsider the Political Power of Female Rage." *New Yorker*, October 8, 2018. https://www.newyorker.com/magazine/2018/10/15/the-perils-and-possibilities-of-anger.

Chahal, Harpreet S., Bizu Gelaye, Elizabeth Mostofsky, Manuel S. Salazar, Sixto E. Sanchez, Cande V. Ananth, and Michelle A. Williams. "Relation of Outbursts of Anger and the Acute Risk of Placental Abruption: A Case-Crossover Study." *Paediatric and Perinatal Epidemiology* 33, no. 6 (2019): 405–411.

Chaplin, Simon. "Anatomy and the 'Museum Oeconomy': William and John Hunter as Collectors." In *William Hunter's World: The Art and Science of Eighteenth-Century Collecting*, edited by E. Geoffrey Hancock, Nick Pearce, and Mungo Campbell, 29–41. New York: Routledge, 2016.

Cheng, Ching-Yu, Eileen R. Fowles, and Lorraine O. Walker. "Postpartum Maternal Health Care in the United States: A Critical Review." *Journal of Perinatal Education* 15, no. 3 (2006): 34–42.

Cheung, Kylie. "Madison Cawthorn, Accused Sexual Harasser, Calls Women 'Earthen Vessels' for Babies." Jezebel, December 6, 2021. https://jezebel.com/madison-cawthorn-accused-sexual-harasser-calls-women-1848166146.

Chicago Museum of Science and Industry. "Prenatal Development." https://www.msichicago.org/explore/whats-here/exhibits/you-the-experience/the-exhibit/your-beginning/prenatal-development/.

Christian, Nicole T., and Virginia F. Borges. "What *Dobbs* Means for Patients with Breast Cancer." *New England Journal of Medicine* 387 (2022): 765–767.

Chrysostom, John. "Homily 24 on Romans." Translated by J. Walker, J. Sheppard, and H. Browne and revised by George B. Stevens. From *Nicene and Post-Nicene Fathers*, First Series, Vol. 11, edited by Philip

Schaff. Buffalo, NY: Christian Literature Publishing, 1889. Revised and edited for New Advent by Kevin Knight. http://www.newadvent.org /fathers/210224.htm

Cicero. *Pro Lege Manilia. Pro Caecina. Pro Cluentio. Pro Rabirio Perduellionis Reo.* Translated by H. Grose Hodge. Loeb Classical Library 198. Cambridge, MA: Harvard University Press, 1927.

Cleveland Clinic. "Am I Pregnant?" https://my.clevelandclinic.org/health /articles/9709-pregnancy-am-i-pregnant.

CNET. "10 Weird Pregnancy Symptoms That Are Totally Normal." August 9, 2021. https://www.cnet.com/health/parenting/weird-pregnancy -symptoms-that-are-totally-normal/.

Cohain, Judy Slome, Rina E. Buxbaum, and David Mankuta. "Spontaneous First Trimester Miscarriage Rates per Woman among Parous Women with 1 or More Pregnancies of 24 Weeks or More." *BMC Pregnancy and Childbirth* 17, no. 437 (2017). https://bmcpregnancychildbirth .biomedcentral.com/articles/10.1186/s12884-017-1620-1.

Coiter, Volcher. *Externarum et Internarum Principalium Humani Corporis Partium Tabulae.* Noribergae, 1573.

Colombo, Realdo. *De re anatomica.* Venice: Nicholas Bevilaqua, 1559.

Commonwealth Fund. "Policies for Reducing Maternal Morbidity and Mortality and Enhancing Equity in Maternal Health: A Review of the Evidence." November 16, 2021. https://www.commonwealthfund.org /publications/fund-reports/2021/nov/policies-reducing-maternal -morbidity-mortality-enhancing-equity#6.

Corriente, Federico. *Dictionary of Arabic and Allied Loanwords: Spanish, Portuguese, Catalan, Galician and Kindred Dialects.* Leiden: Brill, 2008.

Crawford, Patricia. "Attitudes to Menstruation in Seventeenth-Century England." *Past and Present* no. 91 (May 1981): 47–73.

Cunningham, Andrew. *The Anatomical Renaissance: The Resurrection of the Anatomical Projects of the Ancients.* Aldershot, England: Scolar Press, 1997.

Curry, Michael. "Bishop Michael Curry's Royal Wedding Sermon: Full Text of 'The Power of Love.'" NPR, May 20, 2018. https://www.npr.org /sections/thetwo-way/2018/05/20/612798691/bishop-michael-currys -royal-wedding-sermon-full-text-of-the-power-of-love.

D'Alton, Mary E. "Where Is the 'M' in Maternal-Fetal Medicine?" *Obstetrics and Gynecology* 116, no. 6 (December 2010): 1401–1404.

D'Alton, Mary E., Alexander M. Friedman, Peter S. Bernstein, Haywood L. Brown, William M. Callaghan, Steven L. Clark, and William A. Grobman,

"Putting the 'M' Back in Maternal-Fetal Medicine: A 5-Year Report Card on a Collaborative Effort to Address Maternal Morbidity and Mortality in the United States." *American Journal of Obstetrics and Gynecology* 221, no. 4 (2019): 311–317.

Dean-Jones, Lesley. "Menstrual Bleeding According to the Hippocratics and Aristotle." *Transactions of the American Philological Association* 119 (1989): 177–191.

Demaitre, Luke. *Medieval Medicine: The Art of Healing from Head to Toe.* Santa Barbara, CA: Praeger, 2013.

Dembosky, April. "Health Department Medical Detectives Find 84% of U.S. Maternal Deaths Are Preventable." NPR, October 21, 2022. https://www.npr.org/sections/health-shots/2022/10/21/1129115162/maternal-mortality-childbirth-deaths-prevention.

Dickson, Caitlin. "Fetus to Testify against Abortion: A Nine-Week Old Fetus Will Testify before Ohio State's House Health Committee." *The Wire*, March 1, 2011 https://www.theatlantic.com/politics/archive/2011/03/fetus-to-testify-against-abortion/338866/.

Dickson, E. J. "Herbal Abortions Are Going Viral on TikTok. They Could Kill You." *Rolling Stone*, June 29, 2022. https://www.rollingstone.com/culture/culture-news/tiktok-abortion-herbs-misinformation-death-1376101/.

Dioscorides. *De materia medica.* Translated by T. A. Osbaldeston and R. P. A. Wood. Johannesburg, South Africa: Ibidis Press, 2000.

Dobbs, State Health Officer of the Mississippi Department of Health, et al. v. Jackson Women's Health Organization et al. Decided June 24, 2022. https://www.supremecourt.gov/opinions/21pdf/19-1392_6j37.pdf.

Dols, Michael W. "The Origins of the Islamic Hospital: Myth and Reality." *Bulletin of the History of Medicine* 61, no. 3 (1987): 367–390.

Drake, T. G. H. "The Eagle Stone, an Antique Obstetrical Amulet." *Bulletin of the History of Medicine* 8, no. 1 (1940): 128–132.

Dubow, Sara. *Ourselves Unborn: A History of the Fetus in Modern America.* Oxford: Oxford University Press, 2011.

Duden, Barbara. *The Woman Beneath the Skin: A Doctor's Patients in Eighteenth-Century Germany.* Translated by Thomas Dunlap. Cambridge, MA: Harvard University Press, 1991.

Dunstan, G. R., ed. *The Human Embryo: Aristotle and the Arabic and European Traditions.* Exeter, UK: University of Exeter Press, 1990.

Eckholm, Erik. "Anti-Abortion Groups Are Split on Legal Tactics." *New York Times*, December 4, 2011. https://www.nytimes.com/2011/12/05/health/policy/fetal-heartbeat-bill-splits-anti-abortion-forces.html.

Edgar, Amanda Nell. "The Rhetoric of Auscultation: Corporeal Sounds, Mediated Bodies, and Abortion Rights." *Quarterly Journal of Speech* 103, no. 4 (2017): 350–371.

Edgar, James Clifton. *The Practice of Obstetrics*. 4th rev. ed. Philadelphia: P. Blakiston's Son, 1912.

Edwards, Marc. "Fetal Death and Reduced Birth Rates Associated with Exposure to Lead-Contaminated Drinking Water." *Environmental Science and Technology* 48, no. 1 (2014): 739–746.

Eisenberg, Arlene, Heidi E. Murkoff, and Sandee E. Hathaway. *What to Expect When You're Expecting*. New York: Workman, 1996.

Evans, Dabney P., and Subasri Narasimhan. "A Narrative Analysis of Anti-Abortion Testimony and Legislative Debate Related to Georgia's Fetal 'Heartbeat' Abortion Ban." *Sexual and Reproductive Health Matters* 28, no. 1 (2020): 215–231.

Evans, W[illiam]. A[ugustus]. "How to Keep Well: A Plea for Better Maternity Care." *Chicago Daily Tribune*, November 11, 1928, 12. https://archive.org/stream/drevanshowtokeeooevan?ref=ol#page/n13/mode/2up.

Faith2Action. "The Pro-Life Heartbeat Bill." Downloaded January 15, 2022. https://f2a.org/.

Fatima, M., S. Srivastav, and A. C. Mondal. "Prenatal Stress and Depression Associated Neuronal Development in Neonates." *International Journal of Developmental Neuroscience* 60 (2017): 1–7.

Feen, Richard Harrow. "The Historical Dimensions of Infanticide and Abortion: The Experience of Classical Greece." *Linacre Quarterly* 51, no. 3 (1984): 248–254.

Fisher, Mike, and Carrie Underwood. "I Am Second." https://www.iamsecond.com/film/mike-and-carrie/.

Fissell, Mary E. "The Politics of Reproduction in the English Reformation." *Representations* no. 87 (Summer 2004): 43–81.

Flavin, Jeanne. *Our Bodies, Our Crimes: The Policing of Women's Reproduction in America*. New York: New York University Press, 2009.

Flemming, Rebecca. "Galen's Generations of Seeds." In *Reproduction: Antiquity to the Present Day*, edited by Nick Hopwood, Rebecca Flemming, and Lauren Kassell, 95–108. Cambridge: Cambridge University Press, 2018.

Francis, Ellen, Helier Cheung, and Miriam Berger. "How Does the U.S. Compare to Other Countries on Paid Parental Leave? Americans Get 0 Weeks. Estonians Get More than 80." *Washington Post*, November 11,

2021. https://www.washingtonpost.com/world/2021/11/11/global-paid
-parental-leave-us/.

Freedman, Lori R., Uta Landy, and Jody Steinauer. "When There's a
Heartbeat: Miscarriage Management in Catholic-Owned Hospitals."
American Journal of Public Health 98, no. 10 (2008): 1774–1778.

Freidenfelds, Lara. "The Historical Creation and Implications of the
Distinction between Miscarriage and Abortion." Paper delivered at
the American Association for the History of Medicine, 94th Annual
Meeting, May 14, 2021.

Freidenfelds, Lara. *The Myth of the Perfect Pregnancy: A History of
Miscarriage in America.* New York: Oxford University Press, 2020.

Galen. *Galeni De foetuum formatione, edidit, in linguam Germanicam vertit,
commentatus est.* Translated and edited by D. Nickel. Vol. 3, part 3.3 of
Corpus Medicorum Graecorum. Berlin: Akademie-Verlag, 2001.

Gardner, Jane F. *Women in Roman Law and Society.* Bloomington: Indiana
University Press, 1991.

Gellius. *Attic Nights.* Vol. 1, bks 1–5. Translated by J. C. Rolfe. Loeb Classical
Library 195. Cambridge, MA: Harvard University Press, 1927.

Gelman, Lauren. "4 Things That Can Cause a Miscarriage and 4 Things
That Absolutely Can't." *Parents,* October 18, 2022. https://www.parents
.com/pregnancy/complications/miscarriage/what-does-and-doesnt
-cause-miscarriage/.

Gerard, John. *The herball or, Generall historie of plantes.* London: John
Norton, 1597.

Gilbertus Anglicus (Gilbert the Englishman). *Compendium medicine.* Lyon:
Portonaris, 1510.

Gleason, Maud. "Shock and Awe: The Performance Dimension of Galen's
Anatomy Demonstrations." In *Galen and the World of Knowledge,*
edited by Gill, C., T. Whitmarsh, and J. Wilkins, 85–114. Cambridge:
Cambridge University Press, 2009.

Glenza, Jessica. "Doctors' Organization: Calling Abortion Bans 'Fetal
Heartbeat Bills' Is Misleading: American College of Obstetricians and
Gynecologists Says Term Does Not 'Reflect Medical Accuracy or Clinical
Understanding.'" *Guardian,* June 5, 2019. https://www.theguardian.com
/world/2019/jun/05/abortion-doctors-fetal-heartbeat-bills-language
-misleading.

Goldberg, Michelle. "When a Miscarriage Is Manslaughter." *New York
Times,* October 18, 2021. https://www.nytimes.com/2021/10/18/opinion
/poolaw-miscarriage.html.

Graham, Billy. *Hope for the Troubled Heart: Finding God in the Midst of Pain*. New York: Bantam, 1993.

Green, Monica H. "Constantinus Africanus and the Conflict between Religion and Science." In *The Human Embryo: Aristotle and the Arabic and European Traditions*, edited by G. R. Dunstan, 47–69. Exeter, UK: University of Exeter Press, 1990.

Green, Monica H. *Making Women's Medicine Masculine: The Rise of Male Authority in Pre-Modern Gynaecology*. Oxford: Oxford University Press, 2008.

Greenwood, Brad N., Seth Carnahan, and Laura Huang. "Patient-Physician Gender Concordance and Increased Mortality among Female Heart Attack Patients." *Proceedings of the National Academy of Sciences* 115, no. 34 (August 2018): 8569–8574.

Grimes, David A. "The Morbidity and Mortality of Pregnancy: Still Risky Business." *American Journal of Obstetrics and Gynecology* 170, no. 5 (May 1994): 1489–1494.

Grose, Jessica. "After a Miscarriage, Grief, Anger, Envy, Relief and Guilt: There's No 'Normal' Way to Feel after a Pregnancy Loss." *New York Times*, October 2, 2019. https://www.nytimes.com/2019/10/02/parenting/after-a-miscarriage-grief-anger-envy-relief-and-guilt.html.

Grossman, Daniel S., and David J. G. Slusky. "The Impact of the Flint Water Crisis on Fertility." *Demography* 56 (2019): 2005–2031.

Guillemeau, Jacques. *Child-birth, or The Happy Deliuerie of Women Wherein Is Set Downe the Gouernment of Women. In the Time of Their Breeding Childe: Of Their Trauaile, Both Naturall, and Contrary to Nature: And of Their Lying In. Together with the Diseases, which Happen to Women in Those Times, and the Meanes to Helpe Them. To which Is Added, a Treatise of the Diseases of Infants, and Young Children: With the Cure of Them. Written in French by Iames Guillimeau the French Kings Chirurgion*. London: A. Hatfield, 1612.

Gurr, Barbara. "Complex Intersections: Reproductive Justice and Native American Women." *Sociology Compass* 5 (2011): 721–735.

Gurunluoglu, Raffi, and Aslin Gurunluoglu. "Paul of Aegina: Landmark in Surgical Progress." *World Journal of Surgery* 27 (2003): 18–25.

Guttmacher Institute. "State Bans on Abortion throughout Pregnancy." Accessed September 15, 2022. https://www.guttmacher.org/state-policy/explore/state-policies-later-abortions.

Haelle, Tara. "Zuckerberg Helps Destigmatize Miscarriage: These Women Share Their Stories Too." *Forbes*, August 2, 2015. https://www.forbes

.com/sites/tarahaelle/2015/08/02/zuckerberg-helps-destigmatize -miscarriage-these-women-share-their-stories-too/?sh=6ecd7ea03c59.

Haertsch, Emilie. "After Birth." *Lady Science*, March 7, 2018. https://www .ladyscience.com/essays/afterbirth-painmemoir-haer?rq=Haertsch.

Hall, Stephen S. "The Lost Generation: Trump's Environmental Policies Are Putting the Health of American Children at Risk." *Intelligencer*, February 20, 2019. https://nymag.com/intelligencer/2019/02/trump-epa -risking-health-of-american-children.html.

Hankinson, R. J. "Galen's Anatomy of the Soul." *Phronesis* 36, no. 2 (1991): 197–233.

Hansen, Julie V. "Resurrecting Death: Anatomical Art in the Cabinet of Dr. Frederick Ruysch." *Art Bulletin* 78, no. 4 (1996): 663–679.

Hanson, Ann Ellis. "The Eight Months' Child and the Etiquette of Birth: 'Obsit Omen!'" *Bulletin of the History of Medicine* 61, no. 4 (1987): 589–602.

Harkness, Deborah E. "Managing an Experimental Household: The Dees of Mortlake and the Practice of Natural Philosophy." *Isis* 88, no. 2 (1997): 247–262.

Harris-Perry, Melissa V. *Sister Citizen: Shame, Stereotypes, and Black Women in America*. New Haven, CT: Yale University Press, 2011.

Harry Potter and the Chamber of Secrets. Screenplay by Steve Kloves. Warner Bros., 2002.

Harvey, William. *The Circulation of the Blood and Other Writings*. Translated by Kenneth J. Franklin, with an introduction by Andrew Wear. London: J. M. Dent, 1993.

Hasday, Jill Elaine. "On *Roe*, Alito Cites a Judge Who Treated Women as Witches and Property." *Washington Post*, May 9, 2022. https://www .washingtonpost.com/opinions/2022/05/09/alito-roe-sir-matthew-hale -misogynist/.

Healthline. "Weird Early Pregnancy Symptoms No One Tells You About." January 3, 2018. https://www.healthline.com/health/pregnancy/weird -early-symptoms.

Heck, Jennifer L., Emily J. Jones, Diane Bohn, Shondra McCage, Judy Goforth Parker, Mahate Parker, Stephanie L. Pierce, and Jacquelyn Campbell. "Maternal Mortality among American Indian / Alaska Native Women: A Scoping Review." *Journal of Women's Health* 30, no. 2 (2021).

Heipel, Edie. "The *Guardian* Is Wrong: This Is What a 9-Week-Old Unborn Baby Looks Like." *The Catholic World Report*, October 21, 2022. https://www.catholicworldreport.com/2022/10/21/the-guardian-is -wrong-this-is-what-a-9-week-old-unborn-baby-looks-like/.

Hippocrates. *Generation. Nature of the Child. Diseases 4. Nature of Women and Barrenness.* Edited and translated by Paul Potter. Loeb Classical Library 520. Cambridge, MA: Harvard University Press, 2012.

Hirst, Barton Cooke. *A Text-book of Obstetrics.* Philadelphia: Saunders, 1909.

Hoberock, Barbara. "Oklahoma Senate Passes Three Controversial Bills That Would Restrict Access to Abortions." *Tulsa World.* April 21, 2021. Updated May 28, 2021. https://tulsaworld.com/news/state-and-regional /govt-and-politics/oklahoma-senate-passes-three-controversial-bills -that-would-restrict-access-to-abortions/article_82dd32a0-a1f7-11eb -a9b7-ef50630e5134.html.

Holland, Jennifer L. *Tiny You: A Western History of the Anti-Abortion Movement.* Oakland: University of California Press, 2020.

Holland, Kitty. "How the Death of Savita Halappanavar Revolutionised Ireland." *Irish Times*, May 28, 2018. https://www.irishtimes.com/news /social-affairs/how-the-death-of-savita-halappanavar-revolutionised -ireland-1.3510387.

Hopwood, Nick. "Producing Development: The Anatomy of Human Embryos and the Norms of Wilhelm His." *Bulletin of the History of Medicine* 74, no. 1 (Spring 2000): 29–79.

Hurlbutt, Frank R., Jr. "*Peri Kardies*: A Treatise on the Heart from the Hippocratic Corpus: Introduction and Translation." *Bulletin of the History of Medicine* 7, no. 9 (1939): 1104–1113.

Integris Health. "What Is a Food Desert and How Does It Affect the Obesity Crisis in Oklahoma?" August 27, 2019. https://integrisok.com /resources/on-your-health/2019/august/what-is-a-food-desert-and-how -does-it-affect-the-obesity-crisis-in-oklahoma.

Inwood, Brad. *The Poem of Empedocles: A Text and Translation with an Introduction.* Toronto: University of Toronto Press, 1992.

Jarvis, Gavin E. "Early Embryo Mortality in Natural Human Reproduction: What the Data Say." *F1000Research* 5 (November 2016).

Jarvis, Gavin E. "Misjudging Early Embryo Mortality in Natural Human Reproduction." *F1000Research* 9 (July 2020).

Jauhar, Sandeep. *Heart: A History.* New York: Farrar, Straus and Giroux, 2018.

Jimenez, Fidelio A. "The First Autopsy in the New World." *Bulletin of the New York Academy of Medicine* 54, no. 6 (1978): 618–619.

Johannes de Gaddesden (John of Gaddesden). *Rosa anglica practica medicine a capite ad pedes.* Pavia: Girardengis and Birreta, 1492.

Jones, David S. *Broken Hearts: The Tangled History of Cardiac Care.* Baltimore: Johns Hopkins University Press, 2013.

Juvenal and Persius. *Juvenal and Persius.* Edited and translated by Susanna Morton Braund. Loeb Classical Library 91. Cambridge, MA: Harvard University Press, 2004.

Kapparis, Konstantinos. *Abortion in the Ancient World.* London: Duckworth, 2002.

Karant-Nunn, Susan. *The Personal Luther: Essays on the Reformer from a Cultural Historical Perspective.* Leiden: Brill, 2017. See esp. chap. 8, "Martin Luther's Heart," 155–173.

Kassell, Lauren. "Fruitful Bodies and Astrological Medicine." In *Reproduction: Antiquity to the Present Day,* edited by Nick Hopwood, Rebecca Flemming, and Lauren Kassell. Cambridge: Cambridge University Press, 2018.

Kassell, Lauren, Michael Hawkins, Robert Ralley, John Young, Joanne Edge, Janet Yvonne Martin-Portugues, and Natalie Kaoukji, eds. *The Casebooks of Simon Forman and Richard Napier, 1596–1634: A Digital Edition.* https://casebooks.lib.cam.ac.uk/.

Kaufman, M. H. "Frederick Knox, Younger Brother and Assistant of Dr. Robert Knox: His Contribution to 'Knox's Catalogues.'" *Journal of the Royal College of Surgeons of Edinburgh* 46, no. 1 (February 2001): 44–56.

Kellwaye, Simon. *A Defensatiue against the Plague. . . . Whereunto Is Annexed a Short Treatise of the Small Poxe.* London: John Windet, 1593.

Kenny, Stephen C. "The Development of Medical Museums in the Antebellum American South." *Bulletin of the History of Medicine* 87, no. 1 (Spring 2013): 32–62.

King, Helen. "Hippocrates Didn't Write the Oath, So Why Is He the Father of Medicine?" *The Conversation,* October 2, 2014. https://theconversation.com/hippocrates-didnt-write-the-oath-so-why-is-he-the-father-of-medicine-32334.

King, Helen. *Hippocrates' Woman: Reading the Female Body in Ancient Greece.* London: Routledge, 1998.

King, Martin Luther, Jr. "A Tough Mind and a Tender Heart." August 30, 1959. https://kinginstitute.stanford.edu/king-papers/documents/tough-mind-and-tender-heart.

Knoeff, Rina. "Touching Anatomy: On the Handling of Preparations in the Anatomical Cabinets of Frederik Ruysch (1638–1731)." *Studies in History and Philosophy of Science Part C: Studies in History and Philosophy of Biological and Biomedical Sciences* 49 (2015): 32–44.

Knox, Frederick John. *The Anatomist's Instructor, and Museum Companion: Being Practical Directions for the Formation and Subsequent Management of Anatomical Museums.* Edinburgh: Adam and Charles Black, 1836.

Kunstkamera. "Collection Online." http://collection.kunstkamera.ru/en.

Kuriyama, Shigehisa. *The Expressiveness of the Body and the Divergence of Greek and Chinese Medicine.* New York: Zone Books, 1999.

Ladurie, Emmanuel Le Roy. *The Beggar and the Professor: A Sixteenth-Century Family Saga.* Translated by Arthur Goldhammer. Chicago: University of Chicago Press, 1997.

LaVarnway, Jamie, and Effie Craven. "An Overview of Food Deserts in Oklahoma: June 2017." https://www.regionalfoodbank.org/wp-content/uploads/2021/01/Food-Desert-Report-FINAL.pdf.

Lawrence, Susan, and Kae Bendixen. "His and Hers: Male and Female Anatomy in Anatomy Texts for U.S. Medical Students, 1890–1989." *Social Science and Medicine* 35 (October 1992): 925–34.

Lazinski, M. J., A. K. Shea, and M. Steiner. "Effects of Maternal Prenatal Stress on Offspring Development: A Commentary." *Archives of Women's Mental Health* 11 (2008): 363–375.

Leavitt, Judith Walzer. *Brought to Bed: Childbearing in America, 1750 to 1950.* New York: Oxford University Press, 1986.

Lemay, Helen Rodnite. *Women's Secrets: A Translation of Pseudo-Albertus Magnus's De Secretis Mulierum with Commentaries.* Albany: State University of New York Press, 1992.

Leong, Elaine. *Recipes and Everyday Knowledge: Medicine, Science, and the Household in Early Modern England.* Chicago: University of Chicago Press, 2018.

Lewis, J., J. Hoover, and D. MacKenzie. "Mining and Environmental Health Disparities in Native American Communities." *Current Environmental Health Reports* 4, no. 2 (2017): 130–141.

Lind, L. R. *Studies in Pre-Vesalian Anatomy: Biography, Translations, Documents.* Philadelphia: American Philosophy Society, 1975.

Lonie, Iain M. *The Hippocratic Treatises "On Generation," "On the Nature of the Child," "Diseases IV": A Commentary.* Berlin: De Gruyter, 1981.

Lu, Mathew. "Aristotle on Abortion and Infanticide." *International Philosophical Quarterly* 53, no. 209 (March 2013): 47–62.

Lucas, Jessica. "Dangerous Herbal Abortion Misinformation Is Thriving on WitchTok." *Input,* June 28, 2022. https://www.inputmag.com/culture/herbal-abortion-misinformation-tiktok-witches.

Luthra, Shefali, and Abby Johnston. "Texas' Governor Got a Basic Fact about Pregnancy Wrong: When Asked Why the State's New Abortion Restriction Doesn't Provide Exceptions for Rape and Incest, His Answer Misstated What Six Weeks of Pregnancy Really Means." *The 19th*, September 7, 2021. https://19thnews.org/2021/09/greg-abbott-six -weeks-pregnancy-abortion/.

MacDorman, Marian F., Eugene Declercq, Howard Cabral, and Christine Morton. "Recent Increases in the U.S. Maternal Mortality Rate: Disentangling Trends From Measurement Issues." *Obstetrics and Gynecology* 128, no. 3 (2016): 447–455.

Marafioti, Martin. "The Prescriptive Potency of Food in Michele Savonarola's De Regimine Pregnantium." In *Table Talk: Perspectives on Food in Medieval Italian Literature*, edited by Christiana Purdy Moudarres. Newcastle upon Tyne: Cambridge Scholars Publishing, 2010.

Margócsy, Dániel. "Advertising Cadavers in the Republic of Letters: Anatomical Publications in the Early Modern Netherlands." *British Journal for the History of Science* 42, no. 2 (2009): 187–210.

Marmot M. G., G. D. Smith, S. Stansfeld, C. Patel, F. North, J. Head, I. White, E. Brunner, and A. Feeney. "Health Inequalities among British Civil Servants: The Whitehall II Study." *Lancet* 337, no. 8754 (June 1991): 1387–1393.

Marshall, Aaron. "Fetuses to Be Presented as Witnesses before Ohio House Committee Considering Abortion Restrictions." Cleveland.com, March 1, 2011. https://www.cleveland.com/open/2011/03/fetuses_to_be _presented_as_wit.html.

Marshall, Aaron. "Ultrasound Images of Two Fetuses Shown to Lawmakers during 'Heartbeat Bill' Hearing." Cleveland.com, March 2, 2011. https://www.cleveland.com/open/2011/03/ultrasound_images_of_two _fetus.html.

Martin, Nina. "Take a Valium, Lose Your Kid, Go to Jail." ProPublica, September 23, 2015. https://www.propublica.org/article/when-the -womb-is-a-crime-scene.

Martin, Nina, and Renee Montagne. "The Last Person You'd Expect to Die in Childbirth." ProPublica and NPR, May 12, 2017. https://www .propublica.org/article/die-in-childbirth-maternal-death-rate-health -care-system.

Martin, Nina, and Renee Montagne. "Nothing Protects Black Women from Dying in Pregnancy and Childbirth." ProPublica and NPR, Decem-

ber 7, 2017. https://www.propublica.org/article/nothing-protects-black
-women-from-dying-in-pregnancy-and-childbirth.

Martinez, Fidel. "Latinx Files: The Troubling Case of Lizelle Herrera." *Los Angeles Times*, April 14, 2022. https://www.latimes.com/world-nation /newsletter/2022-04-14/latinx-files-lizelle-herrera-release-latinx-files.

Maternal Vulnerability Index. https://mvi.surgoventures.org/.

Mayo Clinic. "Miscarriage." https://www.mayoclinic.org/diseases-conditions /pregnancy-loss-miscarriage/symptoms-causes/syc-20354298.

McClive, Cathy. *Menstruation and Procreation in Early Modern France*. Burlington, VT: Ashgate, 2015.

McClung, Kassie. "Oklahoma Completes First-Ever Report on Maternal Deaths." *The Frontier*, October 23, 2020. https://www.readfrontier.org /stories/oklahoma-completes-first-ever-report-on-maternal-deaths/.

McClung, Kassie, and Brianna Bailey. "She Was Charged with Manslaughter after a Miscarriage. Cases Like Hers Are Becoming More Common in Oklahoma." *Norman Transcript*, January 18, 2022. https://www .normantranscript.com/news/she-was-charged-with-manslaughter -after-a-miscarriage-cases-like-hers-are-becoming-more-common /article_917d6efe-77b9-11ec-8279-97d2fc288815.html.

McCulloch, Alison. "The Rise of the Fetal Citizen." *Women's Studies Journal* 26, no. 2 (December 2012): 17–25.

McKnight, Jenni. "How Carrie Underwood Dealt with Three Heart-breaking Miscarriages." *Hello Magazine*, January 18, 2022. https:// www.hellomagazine.com/healthandbeauty/mother-and-baby /20220118131126/carrie-underwood-heartbreaking-family-loss -miscarriage/.

Meghan, the Duchess of Sussex. "The Losses We Share." *New York Times*, November 11, 2020. https://www.nytimes.com/2020/11/25/opinion /meghan-markle-miscarriage.html.

Mendola, T. S. "Rivers of Babylon: The Story of a Third-Trimester Abortion." *The Rumpus*, January 30, 2018. https://therumpus.net/2018/01 /rivers-of-babylon-the-story-of-a-third-trimester-abortion/.

Meredith, Sheena. *Policing Pregnancy: The Law and Ethics of Obstetric Conflict*. Burlington, VT: Ashgate, 2005.

Mistry, Zubin. *Abortion in the Early Middle Ages c. 500–900*. Suffolk: York Medieval Press, 2015.

Mistry, Zubin. "The Sexual Shame of the Chaste: 'Abortion Miracles' in Early Medieval Saints' Lives." *Gender and History* 25, no. 3 (2013): 607–620.

Mohr, James C. *Abortion in America: The Origins and Evolution of National Policy, 1800–1900*. New York: Oxford University Press, 1978.

Monsivais, Pablo, and Adam Drewnowski. "Lower-Energy-Density Diets Are Associated with Higher Monetary Costs per Kilocalorie and Are Consumed by Women of Higher Socioeconomic Status." *Journal of the American Dietetic Association* 109, no. 5 (May 2009): 814–822.

Monsivais, Pablo, and Adam Drewnowski. "The Rising Cost of Low-Energy-Density Foods." *Journal of the American Dietetic Association* 107, no. 12 (December 2007): 2071–2076.

Morgan, Lynn. *Icons of Life: A Cultural History of Human Embryos*. Berkeley: University of California Press, 2009.

Morris, Theresa. *Cut It Out: The C-Section Epidemic in America*. New York: New York University Press, 2013.

Mulder, Tara. "Ancient Medicine and Fetal Personhood." *Eidolon*, October 26, 2015. https://eidolon.pub/ancient-medicine-and-the-straw-man-of-fetal-personhood-73eed36b945a#.3n2a1fqm3.

Mulder, Tara. "The Hippocratic Oath in *Roe v. Wade*." *Eidolon*, March 10, 2016. https://eidolon.pub/the-hippocratic-oath-in-roe-v-wade-ded59eedfd8f.

Murkoff, Heidi. *What to Expect When You're Expecting*. 5th ed. New York: Workman, 2016.

Musacchio, Jacqueline Marie. *The Art and Ritual of Childbirth in Renaissance Italy*. New Haven, CT: Yale University Press, 1999.

MYA Network. "The Issue of Tissue." https://myanetwork.org/the-issue-of-tissue/.

Najmabadi, Shannon. "Fetal 'Heartbeat' Bill, Which Could Ban Abortions at Six Weeks, Nears Passage in the Legislature. Gov. Greg Abbott, a Republican, Has Signaled That He Is Looking Forward to Signing the Bill." *Texas Tribune*, May 5, 2021. https://www.texastribune.org/2021/05/03/texas-house-abortion-heartbeat/.

Napheys, George H. *The Physical Life of Woman: Advice to the Maiden, Wife, and Mother*. Philadelphia: J. G. Fergus, 1874.

Navajo Birth Cohort Study. https://www.atsdr.cdc.gov/sites/navajo_birth_cohort_study/index.html.

New York Times Editorial Board. "Slandering the Unborn." *New York Times*, December 28, 2018. https://www.nytimes.com/interactive/2018/12/28/opinion/crack-babies-racism.html.

New York Times Editorial Board. "When Prosecutors Jail a Mother for a Miscarriage." *New York Times*, December 28, 2018. https://www

.nytimes.com/interactive/2018/12/28/opinion/abortion-pregnancy-pro
-life.html.

Noor, Poppy. "What a Pregnancy Actually Looks Like before 10 Weeks—In Pictures." *Guardian*, October 19, 2022. https://www.theguardian.com /world/2022/oct/18/pregnancy-weeks-abortion-tissue.

Nowak, Alexandra L., Cindy M. Anderson, Amy R. Mackos, Emily Neiman, and Shannon L. Gillespie. "Stress during Pregnancy and Epigenetic Modifications to Offspring DNA." *Journal of Perinatal and Neonatal Nursing* 34, no. 2 (April/June 2020): 134–145.

Oaks, Laury. "Smoke-Filled Wombs and Fragile Fetuses: The Social Politics of Fetal Representation." *Signs: Journal of Women in Culture and Society* 26, no. 1 (2000): 63–108.

Oklahoma House Bill 2441. http://oklegislature.gov/BillInfo.aspx?Bill=HB2441.

O'Malley, Charles. *Andreas Vesalius of Brussels, 1514–1564.* Berkeley: University of California Press, 1964.

Oster, Emily. *Expecting Better: Why the Conventional Pregnancy Wisdom Is Wrong—And What You Really Need to Know.* New York: Penguin Books, 2013.

Paltrow, Lynn M., and Jeanne Flavin. "Arrests of and Forced Interventions on Pregnant Women in the United States, 1973–2005: Implications for Women's Legal Status and Public Health." *Journal of Health Politics, Policy and Law* 38, no. 2 (April 2013): 299–343.

Pancoast, Seth. *The Ladies' Medical Guide.* 6th ed. Philadelphia: John E. Potter, 1859.

Paré, Ambroise. *On Monsters and Marvels.* Translated and with an introduction and notes by Janis L. Pallister. Chicago: University of Chicago Press, 1982.

Park, Katharine. "The Organic Soul." In *The Cambridge History of Renaissance Philosophy*, edited by Charles B. Schmitt, Quentin Skinner, Eckhard Kessler, and Jill Kraye, 464–484. Cambridge: Cambridge University Press, 1988.

Park, Katharine. *Secrets of Women: Gender, Generation, and the Origins of Human Dissection.* New York: Zone Books, 2006.

Payer, Lynn. *Medicine and Culture: Varieties of Treatment in the United States, England, West Germany, and France.* New York: Henry Holt, 1996. First published 1988.

Pearlin, Leonard I. "The Sociological Study of Stress." *Journal of Health and Social Behavior* 30, no. 3 (1989): 241–56.

Petchesky, Rosalind Pollack. "Fetal Images: The Power of Visual Culture in the Politics of Reproduction." *Feminist Studies* 13, no. 2 (Summer 1987): pp. 263–292.

Phillip, Abby. "Mark Zuckerberg and Priscilla Chan's Refreshingly Honest Facebook Post about Miscarriages." *Washington Post*, July 31, 2015. https://www.washingtonpost.com/news/the-switch/wp/2015/07/31/mark-zuckerberg-and-priscilla-chans-refreshingly-honest-facebook-post-about-miscarriages/.

Pilkington, Ed. "Murder Charges Dropped against Texas Woman for 'Self-Induced Abortion.'" *Guardian*, April 10, 2022. https://www.theguardian.com/us-news/2022/apr/10/texas-woman-murder-charges-dropped-self-induced-abortion.

Platter, Felix. *De corporis humani structura et usu, Liber tertius*. Basel: Froben, 1583.

Pliny. *Natural History*. Vol. 3, bks 8–11. Translated by H. Rackham. Loeb Classical Library 353. Cambridge, MA: Harvard University Press, 1940.

Pliny. *Natural History*. Vol. 6, bks 20–23. Translated by W. H. S. Jones. Loeb Classical Library 392. Cambridge, MA: Harvard University Press, 1951.

Poe, Edgar Allan. "The Tell-Tale Heart." *Pioneer*, January 1843.

Poppick, Laura. "The Long, Winding Tale of Sperm Science . . . and Why It's Finally Headed in the Right Direction." *Smithsonian Magazine*, June 7, 2017. https://www.smithsonianmag.com/science-nature/scientists-finally-unravel-mysteries-sperm-180963578/.

Porter, Janet. "Should Ohio Prohibit Abortions after Six Weeks? YES: We Can't Ignore Universally Accepted Indicator of Life." *Columbus Dispatch*, December 4, 2018. https://amp.dispatch.com/amp/7115261007.

Raglan, Greta B., Sophia M. Lannon, Katherine M. Jones, and Jay Schulkin. "Racial and Ethnic Disparities in Preterm Birth among American Indian and Alaska Native Women." *Maternal and Child Health Journal* 20 (2016):16–24.

Read, Sara. *Menstruation and the Female Body in Early Modern England*. Basingstoke: Palgrave Macmillan, 2013.

Reagan, Leslie J. *When Abortion Was a Crime: Women, Medicine, and Law in the United States, 1867–1973*. Berkeley: University of California Press, 1997.

Receipt book. Unpublished manuscript. [England?], late seventeenth–early eighteenth century. Folger Shakespeare Library. https://luna.folger.edu/luna/servlet (call no. v.b.400 [242]).

Reed, Charles B. *What Every Expectant Mother Should Know*. Girard, KS: Haldeman-Julius, 1924.

[Rhazes]. *A Treatise on the Small-Pox and Measles*. Translated by W. A. Greenhill. London: Sydenham Society, 1848.

Riddle, John M. *Eve's Herbs: A History of Contraception and Abortion in the West*. Cambridge, MA: Harvard University Press, 1997.

Riggs, Damien W., Ruth Pearce, Carla A. Pfeffer, Sally Hines, Francis Ray White, and Elisabetta Ruspini. "Men, Trans/Masculine, and Non-Binary People's Experiences of Pregnancy Loss: An International Qualitative Study." *BMC Pregnancy and Childbirth* 20, no. 482 (2020). https://doi.org/10.1186/s12884-020-03166-6.

Roberts, Dorothy. *Killing the Black Body: Race, Reproduction, and the Meaning of Liberty*. 2nd ed. New York: Penguin Random House, 2017.

Jane Roe, et al., Appellants, v. Henry Wade. 410 U.S. 113. 1973. https://www.law.cornell.edu/supremecourt/text/410/113.

Roosevelt, Theodore. "On American Motherhood." Speech before the National Congress of Mothers. Washington, DC, March 13, 1905. https://nationalcenter.org/ncppr/2001/11/03/theodore-roosevelt-on-motherhood-1905/

Royal College of Surgeons of England. http://surgicat.rcseng.ac.uk/.

Rubenstein, Janine. "Inside Carrie Underwood's Emotional Journey from 3 Heartbreaking Miscarriages to Her Happy Life Now: 'We Are Beyond Blessed.'" *People*, June 19, 2019. https://people.com/parents/carrie-underwood-100-reasons-emotional-journey-miscarriages/.

Rublack, Ulinka. "Pregnancy, Childbirth and the Female Body in Early Modern Germany." *Past and Present* 150 (1996): 84–110.

Salés, Luis Josué. "As Texas Ban on Abortion Goes into Effect, a Religion Scholar Explains That Pre-Modern Christian Attitudes on Marriage and Reproductive Rights Were Quite Different." *The Conversation*, September 2, 2021. https://theconversation.com/as-texas-ban-on-abortion-goes-into-effect-a-religion-scholar-explains-that-pre-modern-christian-attitudes-on-marriage-and-reproductive-rights-were-quite-different-167170.

Savonarola, Michele. *Il trattato ginecologico-pediatrico in volgare*. Edited by Luigi Belloni. Milan: Società Italiana di ostetricia e ginecologia, 1952.

Scarborough, John. "Theodora, Aetius of Amida, and Procopius: Some Possible Connections." *Greek, Roman, and Byzantine Studies* 53 (2013): 742–762.

Schaffir, Jonathan. "Do Patients Associate Adverse Pregnancy Outcomes with Folkloric Beliefs?" *Archives of Women's Mental Health* 10 (2007): 301–304. https://link.springer.com/content/pdf/10.1007/s00737-007-0201-0.pdf.

Sędziwój, Michał. *A New Light of Alchymie: Taken Out of the Fountaine of Nature, and Manuall Experience. To Which Is Added a Treatise of Sulphur: / Written by Micheel Sandivogius: I.e. Anagram Matically, Divi Leschi Genus Amo. also Nine Books of the Nature of Things, Written by Paracelsus, Viz. of the Generations Growthes Conservations Life: Death Renewing Transmutation Separation Signatures of Naturall Things. also a Chymicall Dictionary Explaining Hard Places and Words Met Withall in the Writings of Paracelsus, and Other Obscure Authors. all which are Faithfully Translated Out of the Latin into the English Tongue, by J.F. M.D.* London, 1650.

Sellers, Frances Stead, and Fenit Nirappil. "Confusion Post-*Roe* Spurs Delays, Denials for Some Lifesaving Pregnancy Care: Miscarriages, Ectopic Pregnancies and Other Common Complications Are Now Scrutinized, Jeopardizing Maternal Health." *Washington Post*, July 16, 2022. https://www.washingtonpost.com/health/2022/07/16/abortion-miscarriage-ectopic-pregnancy-care/.

Sharp, Jane. *The Midwives Book, or The Whole Art of Midwifry Discovered. Directing Childbearing Women How to Behave Themselves in Their Conception, Breeding, Bearing, and Nursing of Children in Six Books, viz. . . . / by Mrs. Jane Sharp Practitioner in the Art of Midwifry above Thirty Years.* London, 1671.

Sharp, Sonja. "Post-*Roe*, Many Autoimmune Patients Lose Access to 'Gold Standard' Drug." *Los Angeles Times*, July 11, 2022. https://www.latimes.com/california/story/2022-07-11/post-roe-many-autoimmune-patients-lose-access-to-gold-standard-drug.

Shaw, Steven A. "Chicken of the Sea." *New York Times*, July 15, 2007. https://www.nytimes.com/2007/07/15/opinion/15shaw.html.

Shepherd, Katie, and Frances Stead Sellers. "Abortion Bans Complicate Access to Drugs for Cancer, Arthritis, Even Ulcers: Some Chronically Ill Women Face Questions about Critical Medications That Could Be Used to End a Pregnancy." *Washington Post*, August 8, 2022. https://www.washingtonpost.com/health/2022/08/08/abortion-bans-methotrexate-mifepristone-rheumatoid-arthritis/.

Sheppey, Thomas. A Book of Choice Receipts Collected from Several Famous Authors a Great Part in Monasteries and Often Experimented as to a Great Number of Them. Unpublished manuscript, ca. 1675. Folger Shakespeare Library. https://luna.folger.edu/luna/servlet (call no. v.a.452 [510]).

Simmons-Duffin, Selena. "The Texas Abortion Ban Hinges on 'Fetal Heartbeat.' Doctors Call That Misleading." *All Things Considered*, September 3, 2021. https://www.npr.org/sections/health-shots/2021/09/02/1033727679/fetal-heartbeat-isnt-a-medical-term-but-its-still-used-in-laws-on-abortion.

Siraisi, Nancy G. *Avicenna in Renaissance Italy: The Canon and Medical Teaching in Italian Universities after 1500*. Princeton, NJ: Princeton University Press, 1987.

Siraisi, Nancy G. "Vesalius and the Reading of Galen's Teleology." *Renaissance Quarterly* 50, no. 1 (Spring 1997): 1–37.

Slawson, Shelby. "Heartbeat Act—Open (SS)." Facebook videos, May 19, 2021. https://www.facebook.com/SlawsonForTexas/videos/173245161276116/.

Snyder, Monica. "Guardian Article 'What a Pregnancy Actually Looks Like' Erases Embryos." Secular Pro-Life, October 20, 2022. https://secularprolife.org/2022/10/guardian-article-what-a-pregnancy-actually-looks-like-erases-embryos/.

Solinger, Rickie, ed. *Abortion Wars: A Half Century of Struggle, 1950–2000*. Berkeley: University of California Press, 1998.

Soranus' Gynecology. Translated with introduction by Owsei Temkin. Baltimore: Johns Hopkins University Press, 1956.

Spadaro, Antonio. "A Big Heart Open to God: An Interview with Pope Francis." *America: The Jesuit Review*, September 30, 2013. https://www.americamagazine.org/faith/2013/09/30/big-heart-open-god-interview-pope-francis.

Specia, Megan. "How Savita Halappanavar's Death Spurred Ireland's Abortion Rights Campaign." *New York Times*, May 27, 2018. https://www.nytimes.com/2018/05/27/world/europe/savita-halappanavar-ireland-abortion.html.

Stockman, Farah. "Manslaughter Charge Dropped against Alabama Woman Who Was Shot While Pregnant." *New York Times*, July 3, 2019. https://www.nytimes.com/2019/07/03/us/charges-dropped-alabama-woman-pregnant.html.

Strocchia, Sharon T. *Forgotten Healers: Women and the Pursuit of Health in Late Renaissance Italy*. Cambridge, MA: Harvard University Press, 2019.

Sweet, Victoria. "Hildegard of Bingen and the Greening of Medieval Medicine." *Bulletin of the History of Medicine* 73, no. 3 (1999): 381–403.

Szoch, Mary, ed. *The Best Pro-Life Arguments for Secular Audiences.* Washington, DC: Family Research Council, 2021. https://downloads.frc .org/EF/EF21F56.pdf.

Tacitus. *Annals.* Bks 13–16. Translated by John Jackson. Loeb Classical Library 322. Cambridge, MA: Harvard University Press, 1937.

Taylor, Janelle S. *The Public Life of the Fetal Sonogram: Technology, Consumption, and the Politics of Reproduction.* New Brunswick, NJ: Rutgers University Press, 2008.

Texas Senate Bill 8. https://legiscan.com/TX/text/SB8/2021.

Tikkanen, Roosa, Munira Z. Gunja, Molly FitzGerald, and Laurie Zephyrin. "Maternal Mortality and Maternity Care in the United States Compared to 10 Other Developed Countries." Commonwealth Fund, November 18, 2020. https://www.commonwealthfund.org/publications /issue-briefs/2020/nov/maternal-mortality-maternity-care-us-compared -10-countries.

Tomes, Nancy. *The Gospel of Germs: Men, Women, and the Microbe in American Life.* Cambridge, MA: Harvard University Press, 1998.

Totelin, Laurence M. V. "Sex and Vegetables in the Hippocratic Gynaecological Treatises." *Studies in History and Philosophy of Biological and Biomedical Sciences* 38 (2007): 531–540.

Tsai, Jennifer. "Why We Can't Look Away from Brittney Poolaw's Case." *Bustle,* October 26, 2021. https://www.bustle.com/politics/brittney -poolaw-miscarriage-conviction.

Tucker, Myra J., Cynthia J. Berg, William M. Callaghan, and Jason Hsia. "The Black-White Disparity in Pregnancy-Related Mortality from 5 Conditions: Differences in Prevalence and Case-Fatality Rates." *American Journal of Public Health* 97, no. 2 (February 2007): 247–251.

Tucker, Jennifer. "The Medieval Roots of Todd Akin's Theories." *New York Times,* August 23, 2012. https://www.nytimes.com/2012/08/24/opinion /the-medieval-roots-of-todd-akins-theories.html.

Turk, J. L. "The Medical Museum and Its Relevance to Modern Medicine." *Journal of the Royal Society of Medicine* 87 (January 1994): 40–42.

UC Berkeley. "Center for the Health Assessment of Mothers and Children of Salinas (CHAMACOS) Study." https://cerch.berkeley.edu/research -programs/chamacos-study.

United States Conference of Catholic Bishops. "Respect for Unborn Human Life: The Church's Constant Teaching." https://www.usccb.org/issues

-and-action/human-life-and-dignity/abortion/respect-for-unborn
-human-life.

Valesco de Tarenta. *Practica valesci de tharanta que alias philonium dicitur.*
N.p., 1516.

van de Walle, Etienne. "Flowers and Fruits: Two Thousand Years of
Menstrual Regulation." *Journal of Interdisciplinary History* 28, no. 2
(Autumn 1997): 183–203.

van Diemerbroeck, Ysbrand. *The Anatomy of Human Bodies . . . : To Which
Is Added a Particular Treatise of the Small-Pox and Measles . . .* Trans-
lated from the last and most correct and full edition of the same by
William Salmon. London: Edward Brewster, 1689.

Van Dijck, José. "Bodyworlds: The Art of Plastinated Cadavers." *Configura-
tions* 9 (2001): 99–126.

Vesalius, Andreas. *De humani corporis fabrica libri septem.* Basel: Oporinus,
1543.

Vesalius, Andreas. *On the Fabric of the Human Body. A Translation of De
Humani Corporis Fabrica Libri Septem Book V.* Translated by William
Frank Richardson and John Burd. Carman Novato, CA: Norman Pub,
2007.

Von der Borch, Claudia. "Are Human Remains in Ethically Safe Hands?"
Mummy Stories, April 9, 2020. https://www.mummystories.com/single
-post/are-human-remains-in-ethically-safe-hands.

von Staden, Heinrich. "The Discovery of the Body: Human Dissection and
Its Cultural Contexts in Ancient Greece." *Yale Journal of Biology and
Medicine* 65 (1992): 223–241.

Wailoo, Keith. "The Pain Gap: Why Doctors Offer Less Relief to Black
Patients." *Daily Beast*, April 11, 2016.

Waldman, Ayelet. "On Feeling Like a 'Bad Mother.'" NPR interview
with David Bianculli, June 4, 2010. https://www.npr.org/transcripts
/127403273.

Weaver, Karol K. "'She Crushed the Child's Fragile Skull': Disease,
Infanticide, and Enslaved Women in Eighteenth-Century Saint-
Domingue." *French Colonial History* 5, no. 1 (2004): 93–109.

Webb, Heather. *The Medieval Heart.* New Haven, CT: Yale University Press,
2010.

Weingarten, Karen. "What to Expect When You're Expecting in the
Nineteenth-Century U.S." *Nursing Clio*, October 17, 2019. https://
nursingclio.org/2019/10/17/what-to-expect-when-youre-expecting-in
-the-nineteenth-century-u-s/.

Werber, Cassie. "The 'Dos' and 'Don'ts' of Pregnancy Are Deeply Flawed around the World." *Quartz*, July 28, 2017. https://qz.com/quartzy /1035538/the-dos-and-donts-of-pregnancy-are-deeply-flawed-around -the-world/.

West, Mary M. *Prenatal Care*. 4th ed. Washington, DC: Government Printing Office, 1915.

Westwood, Anthony. *De variolis & morbillis: Of the Small Pox and Measles*. London, 1656.

Wierzbicki, Kaye. "A Cup of Pennyroyal Tea." *The Toast*, May 27, 2015. https://the-toast.net/2015/05/27/a-cup-of-pennyroyal-tea/.

Wilcox, Allen J., Clarice R. Weinberg, John F. O'Connor, Donna D. Baird, John P. Schlatterer, Robert E. Canfield, E. Glenn Armstrong, and Bruce C. Nisula. "Incidence of Early Loss of Pregnancy." *New England Journal of Medicine* 319 (July 1988): 189–194.

Wilcox, W. A. "Poisoning by Pennyroyal." *Boston Medical and Surgical Journal* 78 (1868): 394.

Withycombe, Shannon. *Lost: Miscarriage in Nineteenth-Century America*. New Brunswick, NJ: Rutgers University Press, 2018.

Wolf, Jacqueline. *Cesarean Section: An American History of Risk, Technology, and Consequence*. Baltimore: Johns Hopkins University Press, 2018.

Working, Russell. "Shock Value." *Chicago Tribune*, July 31, 2005. https:// www.chicagotribune.com/news/ct-xpm-2005-07-31-0507310429-story .html.

Wright, Elizabethada, and Mary Fitzgerald. "Performing Bodies: The Construction of the Unconstructed in Gunter von Hagens' Body Worlds." *Survive and Thrive: A Journal for Medical Humanities and Narrative as Medicine* 3, no. 1 (2017): article 12.

Zaimeche, Salah E. "Ibn al-Jazzār." In *The Oxford Encyclopedia of Philosophy, Science, and Technology in Islam*. New York: Oxford Islamic Studies Online, 2014. https://doi.org/10.1093/acref:oiso/9780199812578.001.0001.

Zauzmer, Emily. "Pregnant Carrie Underwood Reveals She Suffered 3 Miscarriages in Last 2 Years." *People*, September 16, 2018. https:// people.com/parents/pregnant-carrie-underwood-3-miscarriages-2 -years/.

Zerbi, Gabriele. *Opus preclarum anathomie totius corporis humani et singulorum membrorum illius*. Venice, 1533.

Zinaman M. J., E. D. Clegg, C. C. Brown, J. O'Connor, and S. G. Selevan. "Estimates of Human Fertility and Pregnancy Loss." *Fertility and Sterility* 65, no. 3 (March 1996): 503–509.

INDEX